Esthetician's Guide
to
Client Safety
& Wellness

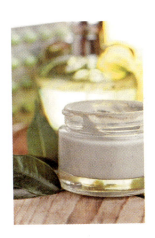

Esthetician's Guide

to

Client Safety & Wellness

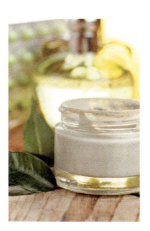

Judith Culp

&

Toni Campbell

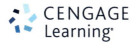

Australia • Brazil • Japan • Korea • Mexico • Singapore • Spain • United Kingdom • United States

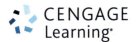

Esthetician's Guide to Client Safety & Wellness
Author(s): Judith Culp and Toni Campbell

President, Milady: Dawn Gerrain

Director of Content & Business Development, Milady: Sandra Bruce

Acquisitions Editor: Martine Edwards

Senior Product Manager: Jessica Mahoney

Editorial Assistant: Elizabeth A. Edwards

Director of Marketing & Training: Gerard McAvey

Senior Production Director: Wendy A. Troeger

Production Manager: Sherondra Thedford

Content Project Management: PreMediaGlobal

Senior Art Director: Benjamin Gleeksman

Title Page Image: © Shebeko/www.Shutter stock.com

For product information and technology assistance, contact us at
Cengage Learning Customer & Sales Support, 1-800-354-9706

For permission to use material from this text or product,
submit all requests online at **www.cengage.com/permissions**.
Further permissions questions can be e-mailed to
permissionrequest@cengage.com

Example: Microsoft® is a registered trademark of the Microsoft Corporation.

Library of Congress Control Number: 2011941745

ISBN-13: 978-1-4390-5745-2

ISBN-10: 1-4390-5745-1

Milady
5 Maxwell Drive
Clifton Park, NY 12065-2919
USA

Cengage Learning is a leading provider of customized learning solutions with office locations around the globe, including Singapore, the United Kingdom, Australia, Mexico, Brazil, and Japan. Locate your local office at: **international.cengage.com/region**

Cengage Learning products are represented in Canada by Nelson Education, Ltd.

For your lifelong learning solutions, visit **milady.cengage.com**

Purchase any of our products at your local college store or at our preferred online store **www.cengagebrain.com**

Visit our corporate website at **cengage.com**.

Printed in United States of America
1 2 3 4 5 6 7 17 16 15 14 13 11

BRIEF CONTENTS

Elena Schweitzer/www.Shutterstock.com

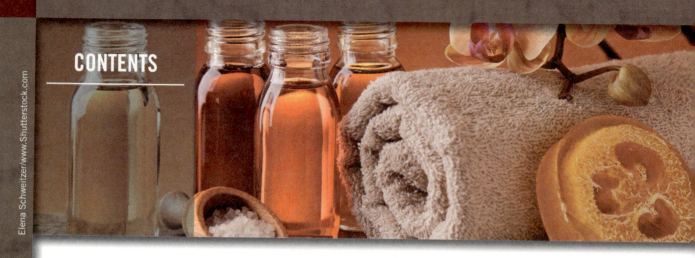

CONTENTS

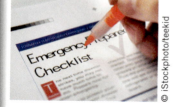

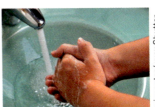

ruigsantos/www.Shutter
stock.com

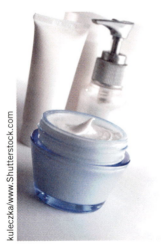

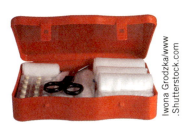

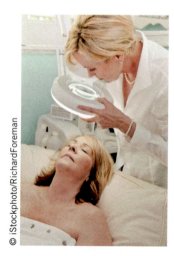

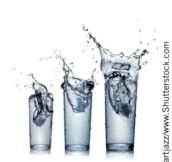

artjazz/www.Shutterstock.com

INTRODUCTION

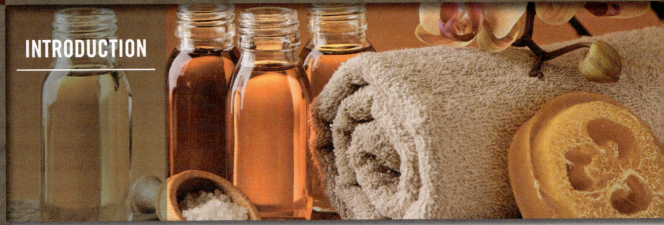

Thank you for obtaining and using the *Esthetician's Guide to Client Safety & Wellness*. By reading this handbook and keeping it nearby as a reference, you are investing in the protection of the health and safety of your clients and yourself. Your clients will appreciate you for the consideration of providing them with a safe experience at every visit. This text will prove useful to you, the esthetician, but may also prevent harm or injury to your clients. Understanding safety and practicing preventative measures is the best deterrent to accidents, injuries and emergencies. However, life and events surrounding us are unpredictable so any manner of unforeseen accident may still occur. Be prepared to be proactive when faced with any obstacle or challenge.

Precautionary measures will decrease the possibility of harm to the client or technician. This handbook provides information on a variety of prevention methods and safety tips. In addition, this handbook provides you with the necessary information of how to best be prepared if faced with an unfortunate injury, accident or emergency situation.

The *Esthetician's Guide to Client Safety & Wellness* is intended for use by future and current practicing estheticians or cosmetologists. No matter how experienced each professional may be questions may arise concerning potential problems. This book is designed to bring a deeper understanding of safety, how to be prepared to work safely and steps to take when you are faced with a new or unexpected situation. During a crisis, many people find it difficult to process information quickly and efficiently in a new or emergency situation. This book will provide the guidance and basis to provide the safest treatments possible. Many simplified step-by-step directions and suggestions for safety checklists are provided for the best course of action. This handbook also provides you with a variety of resource contact information if you feel more support is necessary.

An esthetician is a licensed professional who has a responsibility and obligation to provide assistance to clients or others if needed. In additions to providing assistance to others, information is also provided to increase the personal health and wellness of the professional. By reading this handbook you are investing in your own success.

The intent of this book is not to be considered only advantageous for the advanced professional or the newly enrolled student. Rather this book is designed to be helpful to all levels of experience and in many types of business situations. The primary focus of the *Esthetician's Guide to Client Safety & Wellness* is purely on providing a safe experience for each client and technician. A safe experience for the client is essential to their satisfaction; this safe experience is the basis of providing a feeling of wellness, luxury and relaxation. By investing in this handbook, you are taking a large step toward protecting and assisting yourself and those surrounding you.

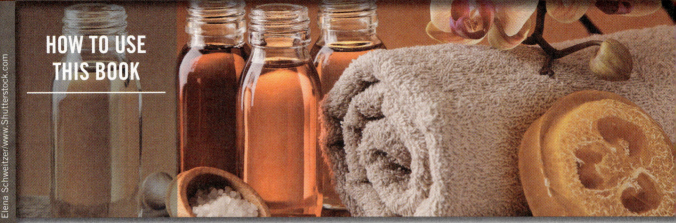

HOW TO USE THIS BOOK

Each chapter of the *Esthetician's Guide to Client Safety & Wellness* begins with a brief introduction of the content provided. The content has been organized and prioritized to ease understanding and avoid confusion. Checklists are provided in applicable chapters, as well as guidelines of instructions for handling different situations. The chapters utilize color coded tabs to allow for easy reference and speedy access. The content has been developed for use as a source of information for future estheticians or for practicing estheticians in the treatment room or as part of a sap operations or safety course.

If a negative or emergency situation were to occur and requires immediate attention, directions are provided to deal with the most common situations. Medications and health concerns come with numerous contraindications or potential safety concerns when paired with certain treatments. A detailed reference to medications and their effects on the skin is provided for you in Appendix A. In addition, contact information for a variety of agencies and associations are provided in Appendix B. This handbook can be an invaluable tool in providing a safe workplace as well as to educate clients on numerous topics of safety and wellness.

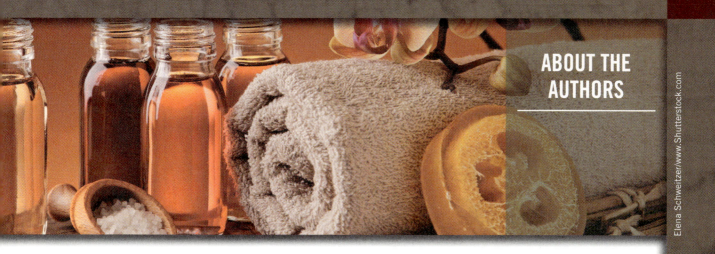

JUDITH CULP

Judith Culp has been an esthetician for over 31 years and has been an employee, an employer and an independent contractor in salons and day spas. She has also been a manufacturer's representative and started teaching advanced skin care classes in the early 1990's. From the time she attended her first trade show, Judith has been "hooked" on education and never been able to get enough. Every year she spends time in continuing education programs and finds something new and exciting in each one she attends.

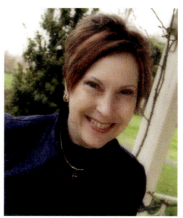

She became Oregon's first CIDESCO Diplomat in 1992 and since then has added NCEA Certification and is a Certified Permanent Cosmetic Professional with the SPCP.

In her career she used her love of teaching first with her clients to help them learn how to achieve their skin care and makeup goals. Then she evolved into teaching advanced classes for a major professional skin care line and her love of teaching took a major leap forward. In 2003 she opened a private career school that taught only esthetics and permanent makeup courses. To meet the need she started writing advanced courses to fill the student's learning objectives. The NW Institute of Esthetics, Inc. now offers programs of 600 and 1200 hours although the state requirements are only 500 hours. She shares with other estheticians via articles in trade magazines, a monthly column in the Stylist and Salon chain and in her work with Milady publishing. She was the subject matter expert for the Milady's Aesthetician Series: Permanent Makeup Tips and Tricks. In 2009 she was the contributing editor for the Milady's Standard Esthetics: Advanced, and is also working in that capacity for the 2nd Edition of this text. Culp is an advocate of continuing education and tries to instill the love of continuing to learn in each of her students. In the midst of a rapidly changing industry, continuing education is critical to the success of the esthetician.

TONI CAMPBELL

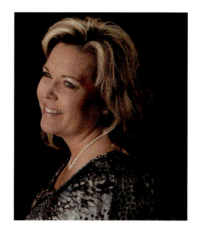

Toni Campbell has been an active professional in the industries of cosmetology, esthetics and education for almost 25 years. Employment in a variety of settings has allowed for a vast amount of experiences to learn from. Campbell has enjoyed learning from the many other professionals she has been able to work with in aspects of skill development, client care and state level curriculum development.

Campbell has enjoyed practicing the development of new learners into professionals for the past 12 years as an educator of cosmetology, nail technology and esthetic disciplines. This portion of her career has placed a primary focus on safety and the instruction of others in safe practices.

Toni Campbell currently is an educator at the secondary level at Sullivan South High School located in Eastern Tennessee. During the minimal spare time, she volunteers her time to assisting the Tennessee State Department of Education in curriculum concerns and works with the national SkillsUSA organization as education chair of the esthetics competitions. Campbell is constantly seeking methods of improving and educating herself with a personal goal of delivering a positive contribution to the industry of beauty and wellness.

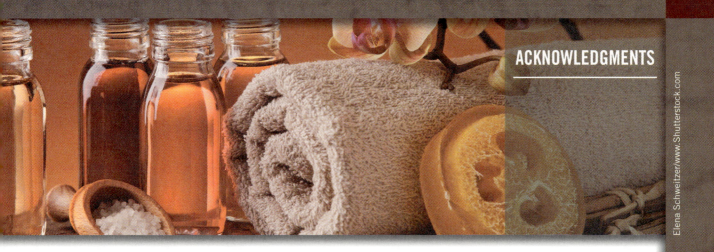

ACKNOWLEDGMENTS

JUDITH CULP

I would like to thank the many people who gave me the opportunity to grow professionally and personally. The esthetics industry is huge in its scope and continues to evolve rapidly. We all have mentors who inspired us to grow and learn. Mine started with the instructor who saw that I obtained the brand new first ever esthetics text book. I cannot thank enough all the industry educators who shared their knowledge and their passion. If they had international certification, well I certainly wanted it too. What I learned in the process is that you never learn it all. Climb one mountain range and another dozen open up before you. I want to thank Cynthia Shaw for believing in my vision of the school focused on esthetics and all of our students over the years who have taught us as much as we have shared with them.

I want to thank Martine Edwards for creating the opportunity of writing this book and to Maria Hebert and Jessica Mahoney for working with me in its development.

A very special thanks goes to Susanne Warfield for her generosity in freely sharing safety information that we were able to include in the book. Also a big thanks to Associated Skin Care Professionals for sharing their client forms. Both resources contributed to making this book more useful and complete.

I also thank the reviewers for their most useful feedback. I value every suggestion that they provided.

Finally, I couldn't have done this without the support of my biggest fan who totally believes in me, my husband Charles.

If you have questions or comments, I welcome your inquiries. You may contact me directly via email: judy.culp@gmail.com. I also have a Facebook page: Judith Culp.

TONI CAMPBELL

I would like to offer my most heartfelt thanks to the many people who have contributed to my opportunity to learn and grow as an esthetician, cosmetologist and educator. Many fellow professionals have provided me with a deeper understanding of skill development and safety and wellness.

I also would like to thank Maria Hebert for opening the door to me as a writer and in the development of this handbook. Maria has always been a pleasure to work with and has provided me with large amounts of insight as well as moral support.

I also thank the reviewers who have so generously provided their time, vision and kindly offered so many suggestions toward the completion of this *Esthetician's Guide to Client Safety & Wellness.*

Ultimately, I could never have accomplished this without the support of my wonderful parents, Don Hickman and Shirley Krell. My beautiful daughters who I love tremendously, Kalleisha (Keisha) and Tallia, and my dear husband who has provided me with moral support and selfless giving of his time; he provides me with all his strength and love resulting in our infinite bond—thank you my precious Scott.

I welcome inquiries from the purchasers of this publication and will be pleased to assist with your questions or comments. You may contact me at stylinteach@hotmail.com

REVIEWERS

The publisher and authors want to thank the following reviewers for their incredibly useful feedback. We appreciate your time and sharing your expertise with us to produce a better product.

Christi Cano: President of Innovative Spa Productions, Henderson, NV.

Suzanne R. Casabella, NYS Licensed Esthetician, Instructor and Program Director, NY

Denise R. Fuller: Port Saint Lucie, FL

Sheilah Fulton: Esthetician/Esthetics Instructor, VA

Laureen Gillis: Kent Career Technical Center, Grand Rapids, MI

Shari Golightly: Director/Instructor/Cosmetologist/CMT/TRM of Entanglements Training Center, Greeley, CO.

Jeanne Valek Healy: Carolina Skin Care Academy, Inc., Columbia, SC

Shelly Hess: Esthetician/Owner, Burbank, CA

Dawn Mango: Instructor at John Paolos Extreme Beauty Institute

Christine Paynter, Director of Education, CO

Beth Phillips: Raymore, MO

Melissa Siedlicki: Clover Park Technical College & Brassfields Salon & Spa, Tacoma, WA

Patricia Powers Stander: Independent Skin Care Consultant, Licensed Esthetician & Esthetics Instructor, Florence, MA

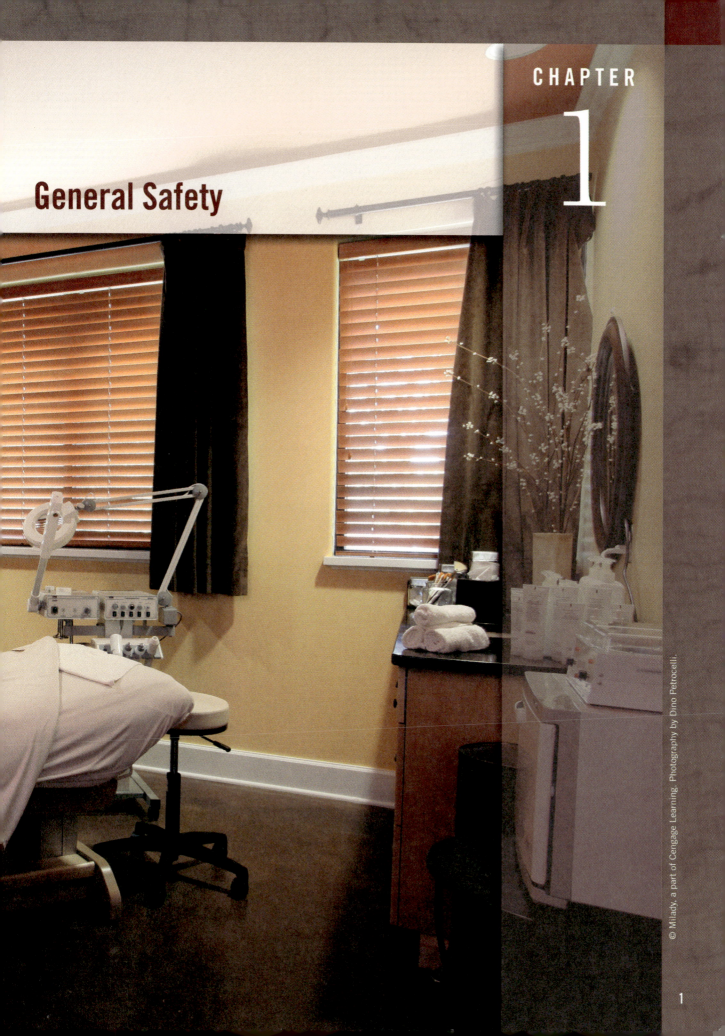

General Safety

INTRODUCTION

Practicing as a licensed esthetician is considered a highly skilled occupation. Clients will place their health and welfare in your hands due to your knowledge, skill and experience. Every client will expect and deserve to receive a safe and satisfying experience while in your care. As a professional, client and technician safety should always be a top priority. To properly practice the highest standards of safety, many components must be diligently practiced on a daily basis. Estheticians must put effort and thought into every service to provide an experience of the ultimate quality. Many components will affect safety habits and must work cohesively in order to ensure appropriate practices are being followed. In this chapter you will find important information concerning professionalism for the esthetician, professional responsibilities, providing client care, and operating in a safe environment.

PROFESSIONALISM

Professionalism can be defined as the quality of possessing the skill, competence, or character of a member of a highly trained profession. Practicing professionalism should be one of your goals and includes a variety of concepts (Figure 1–1). The professional concepts of your overall image, appearance, grooming, and a healthy diet and lifestyle may seem to be unrelated, but when they are incorporated together, they will gain you the respect and confidence of your clients.

Ethics

Practice of professional ethics involves following acceptable moral standards and awareness of how these affect conduct. As a professional, you should always have and follow a basic format of ethical principles; an exceptional guideline of ethical practices specific to your occupation is provided by The National Coalition of Esthetic Association ("NCEA Code of Ethics," n.d.).

NCEA Code of Ethics

- Estheticians will serve the best interests of their clients at all times and will provide the highest quality service possible.
- Estheticians will uphold client confidentiality, maintain treatment and documentation records, and provide clear, honest communication.
- Estheticians will provide clients with clear and realistic goals and results, and will not make false claims regarding the potential benefits of the techniques rendered or products recommended.

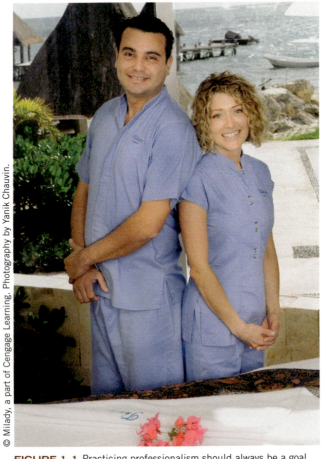

© Milady, a part of Cengage Learning. Photography by Yanik Chauvin.

FIGURE 1–1 Practicing professionalism should always be a goal for the esthetician.

- Estheticians will adhere to the scope of practice of their profession and refer clients to the appropriate qualified health practitioner when indicated.
- Estheticians will offer services only within the scope of practice as defined by the state within which they operate, if required, and in adherence with appropriate federal laws and regulations.
- Estheticians will not utilize any technique/procedure for which they have not had adequate training and shall represent their education, training, qualifications, and abilities honestly.
- Estheticians will strictly adhere to all usage instructions and guidelines provided by product and equipment manufacturers, provided those guidelines and instructions are within the scope of practice as defined by the state, if required.
- Estheticians will follow, at minimum, infection-control practices as defined by their state regulatory agency, the Centers for Disease Control & Prevention (CDC), and the Occupational Safety & Health Administration (OSHA).
- Estheticians will commit themselves to ongoing education and to providing clients and the public with the most accurate information possible.
- Estheticians will dress in attire consistent with professional practice and adhere to the Code of Conduct of their governing board.

The provided code of ethics contains general concepts of ethics that can be applied in many types of establishments. Be conscious that employers, regulations, or the clientele serviced may have more stringent or specific ethical expectations.

Appearance and Image

It is human nature to form opinions about others based on visual appearances. It is therefore of utmost importance that as a professional your appearance always reflect a positive image. How you present yourself to others will affect their perception of your abilities. The most important things to consider in your own image are your personal hygiene and grooming habits. Proper daily hygiene is an indicator that cleanliness is a personal priority. Some factors of your hygiene include practices of daily bathing and use of deodorant; keeping the hair properly cleaned; and regular oral care, including brushing and flossing the teeth daily and regular dental check-ups. Showing concern for your personal appearance and grooming will show that you have pride in yourself and the services you offer. It may seem a troublesome task, but with practice and establishment of a routine, proper hygiene and grooming habits are easily achieved.

Your grooming practices should be appropriate to your workplace and the type of client you provide services to. Elements of your overall appearance include your hair, cosmetic application, and clothing that is worn in a neat and pleasant manner (Figure 1–2). Hair should always be

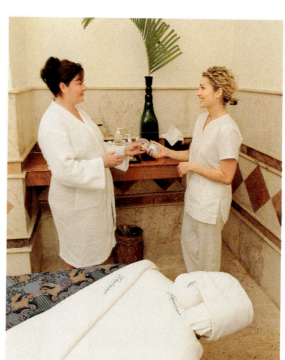

FIGURE 1–2 Grooming habits are a major component of your professional image.

© Milady, a part of Cengage Learning. Photography by Yanik Chauvin.

FYI

Estheticians who wear polish on their fingernails may expose a client to allergic contact dermatitis. An allergic contact dermatitis reaction to nail polish will range from a mild irritation to a severe allergic reaction and commonly occurs on the thin skin of the eyelid.

FYI

Although facial or visible body piercings and tattoos are common in our fashion culture, they may be considered unsightly by some clients and limit your advancement as a professional.

kept clean and neatly groomed; technicians should maintain the style so that hair does not fall into their faces or onto their clients when they lean forward to work. Makeup application should be professional, precise, and not excessive. Many styles of cosmetic application are available but may vary depending on the dynamics of your workplace and the local region.

The hands of an esthetician are one of the most important tools in the performance of esthetic services, and their appearance and hygiene are an essential component of your image. The skin of the hands should be kept unstained and moisturized. Keep the fingernails short, with minimal free edge and smooth, balanced edges. Proper nail length for performing esthetic treatments can be determined by viewing the hand with the palm facing you at eye level: if the free edge is visible, it likely needs to be shortened. Wearing the nails natural is a symbol of freshness and cleanliness; in addition, this practice will prevent contaminants from being hidden in microscopic cracks of polish.

Any jewelry worn while working should be minimal. Any accessories worn while servicing clients should be conservative and must never distract from the service by being bothersome or producing noise. Rings should be smooth so the client's skin cannot be scratched, and necklaces should be short enough so as never to make contact with the client when the esthetician leans forward. Personal choices of clothing should be appropriate for the treatment offerings; many states and employers require that street clothing be covered with various types of uniform wear. Never wear clothing that does not fit correctly or exposes any skin in an inappropriate area. Keep in mind that esthetic treatments may require you to move around throughout a service; clothing may easily gap or sag with your movements. Regular use of lab coats, aprons, scrubs, or other spa attire will help maintain a hygienic environment for treatments. An unsightly and contaminated appearance can be prevented by keeping a clean change of garments available in the event that your clothing becomes soiled during the workday.

Odors and aromas in the treatment room are an important part of the esthetic world. Remember that each client has expectations of a clean and healthy experience while visiting an esthetician, and an unappealing scent may lessen the quality. Technicians should always maintain absolutely fresh breath and have no hint of cigarette smoke on or around them. Since we work in such close proximity to clients, some care must be made with food choices so that post-lunch breath is not a problem. It is worthwhile to keep mints, toothbrush supplies, mouthwash or breath fresheners at work so they are readily available. Never chew gum during consultations or treatments; gum chewing may cause disturbing or distracting sounds or be considered unprofessional. Wearing fragrance or perfume, including the use of scented body lotions and hair products, should be minimal or avoided completely.

Communication

Practicing effective communication is necessary in providing safe treatments to clients. You must be able to convey and clarify important information and address client problems, needs, and concerns (Figure 1–3). It is the responsibility of the esthetician to guide all conversation in the

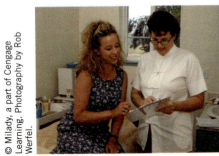

FIGURE 1–3 Effective communication is a necessary part of providing safe treatments.

treatment room. Use of proper communication will create realistic expectations for the client and a thorough understanding of client needs. Clients deserve to know what a service involves and to understand the necessary steps. Our key purpose as estheticians is to help our clients relax and to educate them as to how their skin concerns can be addressed. This means that we need to talk to them as we proceed so that they learn what we can achieve today and what treatments and home-care products will help them achieve their goals.

You may encounter a situation in which a client feels the need to develop a personal relationship with you. It is important to remember that we are not doctors or counselors. Avoid involvement in personal problems or giving advice outside the esthetic scope of practice. Never discuss your personal business with clients and be cautious about topics of conversation, which should never be controversial. Listen quietly and focus on your treatment. You may offer understanding, but avoid becoming emotionally involved. At times you may need to redirect conversation back to that of esthetic concerns or products. Calming, soothing essential oils, chakra stones, Reiki, and music can all be employed to assist the client's emotional state without sacrificing your own well-being. Be certain that proper training has been completed prior to performing treatments involving Reiki and essential oils.

Time Management

An additional component of your professionalism is your time management technique. You should always have respect for a client's time and make efforts to begin each appointment promptly as scheduled. Being organized and prepared in advance for the day ahead will prevent last-minute scrambling to find supplies or to begin a treatment. Advanced planning will allow a client to be escorted to the treatment area at the scheduled time. Skill is also required in client management so that one client does not infringe on time scheduled for another appointment. If a client arrives late, adjustments may need to be made for their treatment so that the technician is not late for subsequent clients. Having a predetermined policy and practicing effective communication skills will prevent client frustration.

CLIENT CARE

Providing optimal care for clients is an important part of addressing safe practices. This begins with the consultation, practicing good communication skills, time management, use of specific leading questions, and providing treatments that will offer a positive outcome.

Consultation

Performing a client consultation correctly is essential to achieving safe and expected results. The technician must gather information in the client consultation process, learning not only about the client's personal skin-care routine, but about health issues, medications, allergies, lifestyle, and any other important factors that may affect the outcome of the treatment. The information obtained during the consultation will alert a technician to any indications, concerns, and contraindications for treatment. The client must also be monitored during the treatment to ensure their comfort and that the procedure is progressing in a positive and safe manner. On the client's first visit, ask them to come 10 to 15 minutes early to fill out the appropriate forms, and schedule a longer appointment for the service to allow for an adequate consultation (Figure 1–4). Depending on the policy of the

Confidential Skin Health Survey

PLEASE PRINT

Today's Date _____

First Name _____ Last Name _____ Date of Birth __/__/____

Street _____ Apt. # _____ City _____ State _____ Zip _____

Phone: Home ( ) _____Work ( ) _____ Mobile ( ) _____

Dermatologist/Physician _____ Phone ( ) _____

Emergency Contact _____ Phone ( ) _____

Your Occupation _____

Referred By ❏ Friend ❏ Mailer ❏ Walk-by ❏ Yellow Pages ❏ Gift Certificate ❏ Other _____

Eesthetician Name _____

1. Is this your first facial? ❏ Yes ❏ No
2. What is the reason for your visit today?
   _____
3. What special areas of concern do you have?
   _____
   _____
4. Are you presently under a physician's care for any current skin condition or other problem? ❏ Yes ❏ No
   What?_____
5. Are you pregnant? ❏ Yes ❏ No
6. Are you taking birth control pills? ❏ Yes ❏ No
   If so, what type?_____
7. Hormone replacement? ❏ Yes ❏ No
   If so, what?_____
8. Do you wear contact lenses? ❏ Yes ❏ No
9. Do you smoke? ❏ Yes ❏ No
10. Do you often experience stress? ❏ Yes ❏ No
11. Have you had skin cancer? ❏ Yes ❏ No

12. Are you now using (or used in the past): ❏ Azelex
    ❏ Differin ❏ Renova ❏ Retin-A ❏ Tazorac
    ❏ Glycolic or alpha hydroxy acids
    If so, when and for how long? _____
13. Are you now using or have you ever used Accutane?
    ❏ Yes ❏ No
    If so, when and for how long? _____
14. Do you have acne? ❏ Yes ❏ No
    Experience frequent blemishes? ❏ Yes ❏ No
    If so, how frequently? _____
15. Do you have any allergies to cosmetics, foods, or drugs?
    ❏ Yes ❏ No
    Please list _____
16. Are you presently taking medications—oral or topical?
    ❏ Yes ❏ No If so, please list.
    _____
    _____
17. What products do you use presently? ❏ Soap
    ❏ Cleansing milk ❏ Toner ❏ Scrub ❏ Mask
    ❏ Creams ❏ Sunscreen ❏ Other

Please circle if you are affected by or have any of the following:

Asthma	Fever blisters	Hysterectomy	Sinus problems
Cardiac problems	Headaches—chronic	Immune disorders	Skin diseases—other
Depression or Anxiety	Hepatitis	Lupus	Urinary or kidney problems
Eczema	Herpes	Metal bone, pins, or plates	
Epilepsy	High blood pressure	Pacemaker	

Please explain above problems or list any other significant issues. _____

I understand that the services offered are not a substitute for medical care and any information provided by the therapist is for educational purposes only and not diagnostically prescriptive in nature. I understand that the information herein is to aid the therapist in giving better service and is completely confidential.

SPA POLICIES

1. Professional consultation is required before initial dispensing of products.
2. Our active discount rate is only effective for clients visiting every 4 weeks.
3. We do not give cash refunds.
4. We require a 24-hour cancellation notice.

I fully understand and agree to the above spa policies.

_____   _____
Client's Signature   Date

FIGURE 1–4 Use of a skin health history form will assist in determining the best treatment for every client.

business, it may be necessary to explain to a client that the consultation time may affect the amount of treatment time, and that the appointment may therefore be adjusted accordingly. Client information must be updated on every visit to the clinic for a service; these updates will alert the technician to any changes that could affect the course of the treatment.

It is essential for each client to be educated in the course of treatments in order to feel the results are desirable. The esthetician must clearly explain to clients the reasons for treatment recommendations and all of the risks, complications, and consequences of the treatment to be performed. It is not uncommon for a client to request an aggressive treatment on a first visit. It is our responsibility as a licensed professional to determine if such a treatment is the best service for them at that point in time.

Case Study

A client comes in on a Friday and wants a chemical exfoliation, often termed a "peel." During the client consultation, the client reveals that he or she has planned a weekend of waterskiing and other outdoor activities. The technician is faced with a safety issue. A chemical peel will increase the skin's sensitivity to the sun and could result in a serious reaction or burn. It is the responsibility of the professional to properly advise the client of the consequences and to recommend a more appropriate treatment (Figure 1–5).

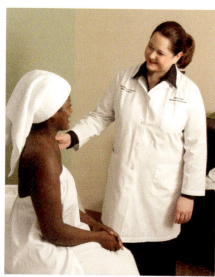

FIGURE 1–5 It is the responsibility of the technician to inform clients of possible consequences.

During the consultation is a good time to have the client sign the appropriate informed-consent forms. This will clarify that you have explained the treatment to them and that the client is willing to follow the appropriate home care and any restrictions that may be associated with their treatment. The informed-consent forms should also include a statement that all responses have been truthful and accurate. A clinic may have one generic form where the details are filled in, but it is more likely there will be specific forms for the treatment to be performed. Some examples of treatments that may have individual and unique directives are waxing, facials, microdermabrasion, exfoliating peels, light therapy treatments, etc. The practice of using written informed-consent forms allows specific post-treatment guidelines to be clarified and easy to follow (Figure 1–6). If special directives are necessary following a treatment, providing the client with written home-care guidelines will result in maximum benefits being achieved. Informed-consent or special home-care directives may be available from product manufacturers, educators, professional associations, or you may need to develop your own.

Interview Questions

Depending on the clinic setup, the client interview may take place in various settings. The location should offer the client a relaxing atmosphere and absolute privacy. The esthetician must allow a client to feel comfortable discussing private confidential information. Some sample

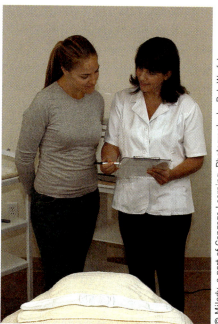

FIGURE 1–6 Always provide clients with written home care guidelines.

questions and points of discussion are listed for you to review during a client intake interview. The client responses will provide the technician with a deeper and more thorough understanding of the precise expectations of the client; every professional may develop his or her own method. The client intake interview should be completed on the initial visit prior to performing any type of treatment.

1. How did you hear about me/us? It is important to determine if the client is a referral, information that can be a useful marketing tool.
2. Have you received a professional facial treatment (or whatever specific service client is requesting) in the past?
3. Describe your prior experience with professional or home treatments (most and least favorite aspects)? The response to this will allow the esthetician to individualize the experience, resulting in the most pleasant experience possible for the client.
4. What specifically are your concerns today? These client concerns offer a technician guidance in how to best help a client and meet their goals ensuring a more positive result.
5. Review medical conditions, discussing any details that might be of concern for the service with client. This discussion of client health will assist in the recognition and prevention of negative results.
6. Review all client medications, including over-the-counter drugs. Discuss all medications that might be of concern or a contraindication with client treatments in order to prevent problems from arising. A technician uncertain about a drug's side effects or contraindications can look it up in a pharmacology drug reference book or in one of the on-line medication reference websites.
7. Ensure that all supplements and herbal remedies are listed and reviewed in addition to medications. Some supplements can have strong effects on the body and make the client more prone to bruising or more photosensitive.
8. Ask if the client has undergone any recent (within the past year) medical procedures. If the client has undergone any, discuss the type of treatment and when it was received. Discuss if the client has been released to resume all normal activities. All responses assist in determining whether requested treatments are appropriate for the client.
9. Discuss any past injuries that may compromise the client's ability to get on and off the facial lounge safely or to be comfortable during a treatment. If the client is in pain from another condition, the treatment may not be appropriate for him or her.
10. Does the client have any product allergies or sensitivities that the technician should be aware of? This feedback helps the technician choose the best product and ingredient selections.
11. Determine if the client has a favorite aroma or if there are specific scents that the client is sensitive to. The impact of odors, aromas, or fragrances can be profound, so it is critical to be informed of client preferences.
12. Request information of current client conditions of pregnancy or lactation. This is critical information and is a safety and liability issue for some procedures and or clients.

FYI

If warranted, do not leave your client unattended in the treatment room. Assist your client on and off the facial lounge.

Treatment-Specific Questions

Depending on each situation and the individual client, the esthetician may need to ask a different type of question or request other information. Some examples of additional discussions or questions are provided for you.

1. Have your medications or health changed since your last visit? The client may now be taking a prescribed medication that could have a negative impact for specific treatments. Blood thinners, antibiotics, seizure medications, and strong pain medications could all impact the client and their treatment.
2. What has been your UV exposure in the past week? Pre- and/or post-treatment exposure to UV rays can cause hyperpigmentation for some services such as peels, microdermabrasion, or waxing.
3. What are your plans for the next few days? This tells us about social obligations, travel, outdoors activities, and other types of events that the treatment could impact or be impacted by.

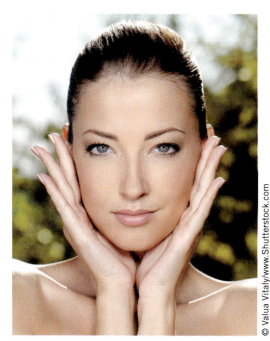

FIGURE 1-7 Client who is pleased with previous treatments.

4. When did you last use any anti-aging topical product, what type of product is it, and how is it used? These are safety questions to establish the appropriateness of the treatment scheduled for today.
5. Have you had any cosmetic injectables in the last four months? What and when? Working on a client with very recent injectables could cause negative effects of the injectables or increase the rate of skin absorption. It is important to know as much as possible about what is implanted in the skin so that treatments have positive outcomes. A client may also be more prone to bruising in the treated area for the first 10 to 14 days following injections.
6. Ask clients to describe how they felt about the results of their last esthetic treatment. Were they pleased or disappointed? (Figure 1–7) Do they wish to add, delete, or change any portion of the treatment?

STATE REGULATORY ALERT

The United States government has federal privacy standards to protect patients' medical records and health information. These laws must be followed in all medical settings, including skin-care clinics and medical spas. HIPAA, the Health Insurance Portability and Accountability Act of 1996, is meant to protect individuals with regard to obtaining information about their health. This means that clients or patients visiting a medical spa or clinical skin-care facility may file a formal complaint about a practitioner who breaches their confidentiality. Estheticians working in these settings should be aware that can be held liable for sharing information about others and should be cautious to never discuss clients or patients with others (U.S. Department of Health and Human Services, 2003).

PROFESSIONAL RESPONSIBILITIES

Compliance with all federal and state regulations is the ultimate responsibility of the esthetician and is also expected by insurance coverage. Professionals must attend continuing education classes, seek out updates to regulations, and be certain they comply with all regulations. Otherwise, they will be bringing great risk to themselves and their clients. It is the responsibility of the licensed professional to offer clients highly skilled techniques safely; never perform any service until appropriate training has been received. It is also imperative for the esthetician to complete and maintain proper documentation correctly and in accordance with regulations.

Procedural Techniques

Many techniques practiced by an esthetician must be approached with consideration for the client. A client should never feel uncomfortable or ill at ease. As long as clients feel safe and secure, they will be more likely to communicate openly with technicians. Being properly trained and prepared in advance will show that you have a high regard for client protection.

When using new or different products, be certain to research the ingredient list and instructions for product use. Never use any product without seeking detailed information in advance; requesting the Material Safety Data Sheet (MSDS) is a great place to begin. Always read the instruction manual provided by the manufacturer when new equipment has been purchased (Figure 1–8). Even when equipment is being replaced, the manual may contain updated and more current information. Completing registration with a manufacturer will provide the company a method of contacting you in the event of equipment safety changes or recalls. Always keep all safety manuals in an organized filing system in case they are needed for future reference.

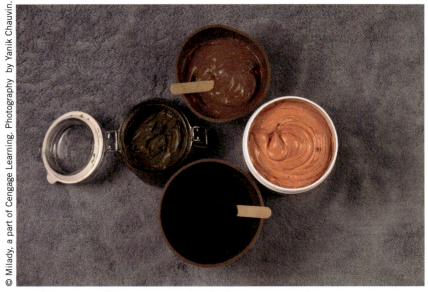

© Milady, a part of Cengage Learning. Photography by Yanik Chauvin.

FIGURE 1–8 Research the use of all equipment and the ingredients list of all treatment products.

Some of the services that estheticians offer, such as bikini or Brazilian waxing, deal with intimate areas of the body. An esthetician who wears gloves while working, offers the client disposable underwear, and provides privacy towels allows a client to feel more comfortable. Maintaining a professional attitude, demeanor, and conversation are critical for instilling client confidence and will prevent feelings of unease or distress.

Following the highest standards of safety to prevent any cross-contamination are visual impacts the client will remember and share. If the client seems concerned, technicians should explain all methods of cross-contamination prevention being used. A client will remember small details such as if pressure is too light or too heavy, towels too hot or cool, equipment malfunctions, and the myriad of other little details that are part of professional techniques.

At all times clients must be made to feel confident that they are being cared for and in the hands of a true professional. Be perceptive to your client and look for any indications of apprehension or discomfort.

Documentation and Recordkeeping

Client documentation and recordkeeping is required by regulatory agencies and insurance providers. Failure to practice proper documentation will place the client and technician at risk. Some states dictate that certain minimal required information be recorded, as well as how long it should be maintained. Some areas may leave it for the technician to determine what is necessary. Vital documents include a client history/lifestyle form, treatment-specific notes, and informed consent with appropriate home care directions. Before and after photographs can be very helpful and are becoming a more commonly used tool (Figure 1–9). This is especially useful when a series of treatments is being performed, so that you may visually monitor improvements.

Using a consent form is strongly suggested and may be required with some services. With the diversity of treatments being offered, a single form may not be adequate. If a single form is used, there must be adequate blanks so that the details of the treatment can be spelled out as well as specific home care. The client should either receive a copy of this form or a separate handout that documents that the client has been provided specific follow-up instructions. The necessary content of forms will be dictated by the services offered at a facility; additional specific information may be provided for treatments such as post-peel, post-waxing, post-microdermabrasion, post-laser (or Intense Pulsated Light [IPL]) hair

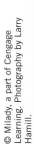
© Milady, a part of Cengage Learning. Photography by Larry Hamill.

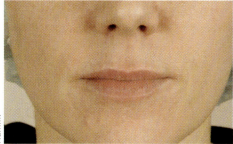 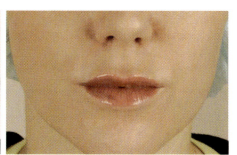

FIGURE 1–9 Before and after photos, such as this lip augmentation, are helpful visual aids.

removal or facial rejuvenation, post-body treatments, etc. Check with manufacturers and your insurance provider for suggested consent and post-care forms.

SOAP Notes

SOAP notes are a method or format of documentation utilized by health care providers. The SOAP note format addresses important information that is then recorded in a particular order. This helps simplify the process and improve the facilitation of treatments. Becoming familiar with this format will help an esthetician develop superior recordkeeping habits. The acronym SOAP stands for subjective, objective, assessment, and prognosis or plan.

- S – Subjective. This is what the client says. Note this using the client's words.
- O – Objective. This is what you observe upon client examination.
- A – Assessment. This is putting in writing your determination of the appropriate treatment and the details of that treatment.
- P – Prognosis or plan. This is your plan or recommendations for client home care, future treatments or referrals to another professional.

Begin this format of documentation prior to the treatment and make additions as needed. During and after the treatment, document exactly what was done and the results, noting any skin reactions, improvements, and client comments. In cases of litigation, technician notes can be critical for validating what was done and the result. When making these notes, keep to the facts and avoid unnecessary clutter. Avoid personal opinions or emotion-based comments; these could be difficult to deal with if the notes were ever subpoenaed in a litigation case. Reviewing the provided sample scenarios may help you with mental organization of SOAP note use.

Case Study

A client requests a treatment with the expectation of unachievable results (e.g., removal of age spots, telangiectasia, and wrinkles in the day's facial). We note this in our assessment and then in prognosis note that we are referring them to a medical professional for evaluation and perhaps medical treatments.

Case Study

A client comes in for a treatment wishing to address skin discoloration and roughness and signs of aging. We observe from skin typing scales that the conditions present are uneven skin tone and some hyperpigmentation, dehydration, and fine lines. We note these observations then perform a hydrating, exfoliating treatment, detailing the steps in assessment. During the treatment, we discuss with the client the required home care to work toward their goals and a series of treatments to address the skin conditions (Figure 1–10). These are noted in our future plan. The client is pleased with the treatment, agrees to our plan, and schedules a series of treatments. We document this information along with products purchased.

The more specific and detailed notes are, the easier it will be to follow a plan and assist the client in achieving their goals. While it may not seem hard to remember what you are doing for a client, it is critical to establish this habit so that quality of services can be maintained as your client base increases. It is also helpful in cases where more than one esthetician may be offering treatments to a client; this commonly occurs in a setting where there are multiple technicians working.

GENERAL ENVIRONMENTAL SAFETY

Once you have a strong understanding of the necessary components of maintaining yourself as a professional and your client-care responsibilities, you should consider the treatment setting or environment. Every salon, spa, or clinic environment should always be maintained in a safe and clean manner. Begin by entering the clinic and looking around carefully as a new client would. Continue to move through all the different areas of your business space. Try to list any possible safety concerns as you proceed. It can be a difficult task to try to foresee any potential safety hazards in a familiar environment. You may need to request assistance from a friend, family member, or possibly a student in esthetic training; this will provide a fresh perspective on the environment. Try to list as many types of potential safety concerns or questions as possible. After you have gathered the information, you may organize it and use the content to design a personalized safety checklist. Always remember that it is essential for a professional to provide an environment with no risk of injury to clients, employees or other visitors (Figure 1–11).

Ergonomics

Ergonomics is the practice of adapting work conditions to suit the worker; practicing ergonomics will result in a safer and more comfortable work environment. Repetitive movements and unnecessary stretching may be the cause of muscle strain and tiring. Ensure that equipment and body position are maintained for proper spine and body alignment. Some examples of how to practice proper ergonomics are provided for you here.

- Align the technician stool with the facial chair for the best height and position for performing treatments.
- Adjust the height of the technician stool as needed.

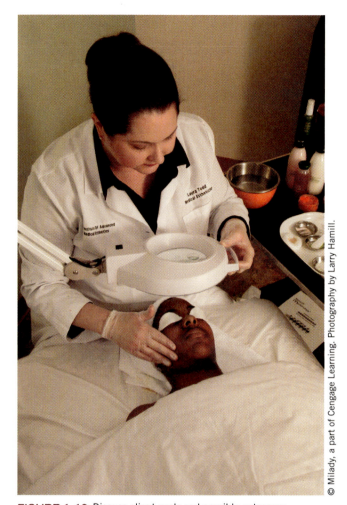

FIGURE 1–10 Discuss client goals and possible outcomes.

© Milady, a part of Cengage Learning. Photography by Larry Hamill.

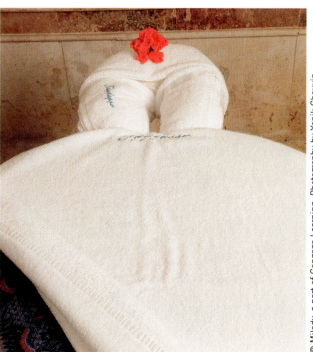

FIGURE 1–11 Always maintain treatment areas in safe and clean condition.

© Milady, a part of Cengage Learning. Photography by Yanik Chauvin.

- Place both feet flat on the floor while seated.
- Adjust the workspace to allow the hands of the technician to remain below chest level.
- Arrange the supply cart or countertop as close as possible to avoid excessive reaching.
- Stand up if something is not in close reach or to adjust equipment.
- Be aware of the position of your posture and back; remind yourself to sit up straight.
- Regularly stretch and loosen the hands and wrists to maintain flexibility.

Safety Checklist

In the clinic setting, the easiest way to achieve a safe environment is by reviewing a checklist of important and common issues and techniques. This will help to ensure that nothing is overlooked and that a safe environment is provided for both client and technician. Making time to develop one or more checklists will prevent hurried or neglectful mistakes in the future. Overlooking even a tiny detail could compromise a safe environment.

You may establish checklists to fit individualized needs and ensure that daily, weekly, monthly, and quarterly housekeeping is performed. Your checklist may vary depending on the treatments or services offered. Opening and closing checklists are helpful for ensuring that infection control and safety goals are achieved, and smaller checklists may be developed for individual treatment rooms or equipment. Checklists should be developed specific to every clinic and should be based on the floor plan, equipment used, treatments offered, and business needs of each clinic. Some general guidelines when developing checklists are to keep listings short and specific, and to organize according to area.

Do not expect checklist development to be a quick and simple task. Checklists will need regular reviewing and updating. Upon beginning the checklist criteria, prioritize the list based on amount of use. From the prioritized list, begin with daily needs of the clinic and then use the remaining criteria to develop a checklist for weekly, monthly, quarterly, and yearly reviews. Operating a safe environment should be a top priority at all times for everyone and will involve a wide range of factors. Deciding to operate in a safe environment is a responsible and conscientious decision. This is necessary to protect our own health as well as that of staff and clients. Provided are some additional ideas and questions for you to consider, but you should continuously ask yourself, "Is there anything else that could be a safety hazard?" and make adjustments to your checklist.

Traffic Areas

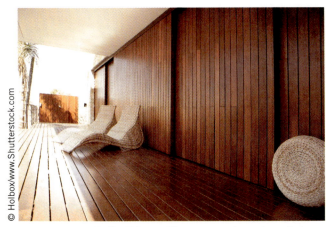

FIGURE 1–12 Verify all foot traffic areas are clean, dry and clear of any obstacles.

- Keep all traffic areas clear, clean, and dry. Are there any barriers that could block movement through the clinic (Figure 1–12)?

- Check that all floors and walkways are safe. Prevent tripping hazards by securing any rugs and ensuring that tiles have no raised corners and no boxes or shelving create obstacles. Immediately and thoroughly clean and dry any spills or products on floors. If working in an environment where flooring may become wet, provide drainage, rubber mats, or slip-free footwear.
- Are all cords, boxes, shelving, and furnishings placed out of the direct flow of traffic?
- Assess the entryway for ease of access, with a freely opening door. Check thresholds and steps for tripping hazards and provide a doormat if needed.
- If the facility is not located on the ground floor, can it be easily accessed by clients, staff, and delivery persons without risk of injury?

Infection Control

- Maintain all areas in a sanitary condition. Consider the reception area, hallways, treatment rooms, and restrooms. Are all work surfaces clean and ready to use? Are drawers, cabinets, and storage areas clean?
- Utilize all standards of infection control. Are appropriate disinfectants available, do they meet state requirements, and are appropriate standards being followed for their use? Are all implements properly cleaned, disinfected, and stored, or properly discarded? Are there written requirements for all technicians to follow OSHA and CDC guidelines of infection control? This will include hand washing, protective equipment such as gloves or face masks, and proper disposal of any sharps.
- Are trash receptacles ample, sufficiently covered, and placed out of the way?
- Provide sharps containers in every treatment area. Check for fill level and arrange for replacement and removal of used sharps as necessary.
- Maintain adequate stock of all personal protective equipment so it is readily available.
- Are restrooms clean, supplied, and in good working order?
- Is each treatment room clean, supplied, and in good working order?
- Are proper standards for washing of linens being followed? Are clean linens properly stored?
- Are disinfectant solutions in the container mixed and changed following the manufacturer's guidelines and regulations? Do all disinfectants have an EPA (Environmental Protection Agency) number to verify proper testing has been done?
- Follow all local and state guidelines for disinfection. If none are defined, follow OSHA and CDC guidelines, as these are national and must be followed unless a state has stricter standards.

Electrical Hazards

- Remove all plugs by pulling on the plug, not the cord.
- Check all equipment before use for cracks in electrical cords and never allow cords to become bent or twisted.

STATE REGULATORY ALERT

States and cities vary in their requirements for the removal of full sharps containers and other biohazards. It is important to check local requirements for proper disposal and follow these guidelines. Providers of public sanitation removal services or medical supply distributors may be helpful with this information or the contact number for the appropriate business that handles this.

- Check that prongs of electrical cords are unbent and plug housing and cord connections are secure for safe operation.
- Check all outlets to ensure no overloading is occurring and that cords are covered in a manner to ensure safe traffic flow and prevent tripping and falling hazards.
- Use only UL- (Underwriters Laboratories), CE- (Conformance European), or CSA- (Canadian Standards Association) listed equipment (Schmaling, 2009).
- Ensure that an adequate electrical supply is in place for the equipment to be used. This will avoid overloading of circuits (Figure 1–13).
- Check that the fuse box is accessible if needed and has a securely closing metal door.
- Never handle electrical equipment with wet hands and never clean equipment while it is plugged in.

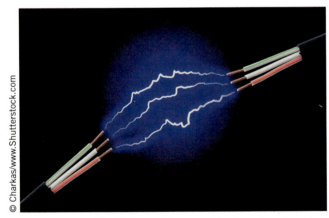

FIGURE 1–13 Electricity must be a consideration of a safe work environment.

Plumbing

- Check the thermostat on the hot water heater. Most experts recommend that hot water temperature should not exceed 125° F (51.66° C). Any water temperature exceeding this poses serious risk of burns.
- Check that all water faucets function properly without leaks.
- View that all drainage systems are not clogged and will efficiently drain.
- Check for proper water pressure and have a pressure valve installed if necessary.
- Water filtration systems may be needed in your area. It is recommended that some form of drinking water be available for clients and your facility may need a filtration system (Figure 1–14). Though it is unlikely, local water supplies can still be contaminated from naturally occurring minerals and chemicals, bacteria, viruses and parasites, or industrial causes.

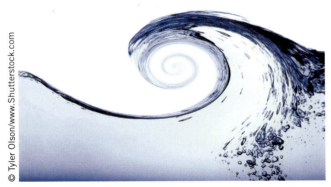

FIGURE 1–14 A water filtration system may be necessary to provide water free of chemicals and minerals.

- Maintain an adequate method of providing distilled water for steamers.

Lighting

- Check that lighting is sufficient and all areas are clearly visible. Replace bulbs as needed.
- View that all light switches are in proper operating condition.
- Are all lighting fixtures securely in place and do any need cleaning?

Signage/Walls

- Check walls for safe condition. Are there any exposed nails or splintered edges of moldings? If any walls are moveable, can they be securely locked into place?
- Post signs that are clearly labeled, easy to view, and simple to understand. This may include signs on exits, doorways to treatment rooms, restrooms, and storage or dispensary areas.
- Is the facility properly licensed and are all required licenses properly posted? Are all practitioners properly licensed, and are those licenses properly displayed?
- Check that all exit doorways are clearly labeled and easy to find.

Ceilings

- Ensure that all ceilings are secure with no risk of falling plaster or tile.
- Check ceilings for any leaks and pay attention to any roof concerns so they may be reported or repaired.
- If a sprinkler system is installed, check to be certain that no sprinkler heads or pipes are painted over, blocked, or covered. Have regularly scheduled checks by a professional to ensure the system is working properly.

Air Quality

- Check for air quality. Are odors and vapors filtered? Is there a ventilation system to provide fresh air? Is regular maintenance necessary?
- Is there any concern about common air problems, such as radon or molds, in your facility?
- Are air filters cleaned or replaced on a regular basis? Do ceiling vents need to be cleaned from collections of dust?
- If windows are used, do they open and close easily? Is the outside air quality satisfactory for a clinic environment?

Equipment/Furnishings

- Check that all furnishings are placed to allow the technician to practice proper ergonomics (Figure 1–15).
- Check all equipment and supplies prior to use to ensure safe operations. Is equipment clean and in good repair?

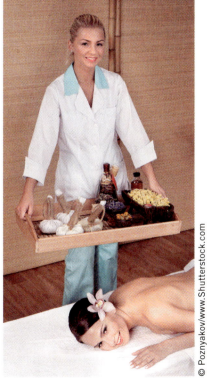

FIGURE 1–15 Place all furnishings to allow use of proper ergonomics.

© Poznyakov/www.Shutterstock.com

- Make sure no nuts, bolts, knobs, or fittings on the facial lounge have worked loose and that all components are functioning properly.
- Check the magnifying lamp to make sure knobs and adjustors are working properly.
- Check that the steamer is properly maintained and operational.
- Has equipment for microdermabrasion, ultrasonic, galvanic, and so forth been checked and confirmed operational?
- Ensure that all elements of the waxing unit are clean and free of wax. The wax should be turned on upon arrival so that it will be ready for the first client. A lid or tent of foil should be placed over the pot to protect contents from airborne particles. Wax turned on high to heat should never be left unattended.
- Is the treatment bed set up properly for the service to be offered, with all components clean and meeting the criteria for prevention of cross-contamination?
- Check devices to be used to determine whether they are functioning properly.

Storage Areas

- Cabinet doors in treatment rooms should open and close properly and have child locks installed if necessary. Ensure that all cabinets are secured to walls and that interior shelving is sturdy.
- Are all linen supplies clean and properly stored to prevent contamination?
- Check that all general storage areas have secure shelving and that items are stored correctly.
- Maintain the dispensary in a clean and orderly fashion. Never place heavy items on high shelving, and use a separate area for food and drink storage or consumption.

Safety Planning

Some key questions to consider in developing a business or personal safety checklist and planning are provided for you:

- Is a written safety plan for emergency situations, including emergency providers' contact numbers, stored in a central location?
- Update CPR, first-aid, and bloodborne pathogen information annually. Did you check that all necessary supplies are replaced as needed and that items are not expired?
- Did you create clinic safety standards and protocols and update them at least annually?
- Have a binder with all MSDS forms in a specified location that will be easily accessible. Are MSDS files organized and kept up to date?
- Is there a system for documenting and storing a report on an incident? Is a system in place for dealing with client or staff concerns and issues?
- Are safety protocols for chemical use, storage, and disposal in place and being followed?
- Is personal protective equipment for each procedure documented? Is it being used? Are adequate supplies of personal protective equipment

such as gloves and safety glasses available? Are staff trained and following guidelines for their use?

- Are adequate quantities of disposable client supplies available? Are staff following proper guidelines for their use?
- Is a safety program in place to deal with a client or staff member accident or illness?
- Are all staff members up to date in their CPR, AED, and first-aid training? Are all staff up to date on infection control and bloodborne pathogen training?
- Are all first-aid supplies available and complete?
- Is a plan in place to deal with emergency situations that require a medical professional or emergency care?
- Is the facility equipped with adequate fire extinguishers, and are these current in their recharging? They need to be checked and recharged annually. Are staff trained in the proper use of fire extinguishers and emergency evacuation?
- Are there protocols in place to guide staff in the event of a natural disaster or storm such as a hurricane, tornado, flood, or earthquake? Are staff trained and current on these protocols?
- Is your facility required to have a fire inspection? Would you pass if it were inspected?
- If a health inspector were to visit, would the facility meet standards for cleanliness, and health and safety guidelines?
- Is there a protocol for the handling of body fluids in case of an accident or injury? Are all staff trained in this protocol?

Client Care/First Aid

- Does every client receive a thorough client intake interview? If a repeat client, ensure that there have been no changes that could affect treatment outcome. Are the proper forms filled out correctly and completely?
- Review client record cards for important information. Any necessary additions can be requested on future printing orders. Are proper client treatment records being documented and stored?
- Are there protocols in place for client product reactions? Are staff trained in these?
- What provisions have been made for flushing the eyes in case of irritation?
- Do all products meet freshness criteria (Figure 1–16)? Products should always look fresh, have no rancid odors or discoloring, and meet shelf-life dates.
- Consider whether professional relationships have been developed with local health care providers. These can be beneficial in the event a client needs referral.

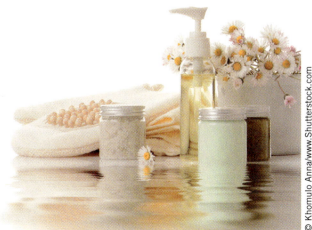

FIGURE 1–16 Ensure all products meet freshness criteria for optimal client care.

© Khomulo Anna/www.Shutterstock.com

- Are there guidelines in place for proper ergonomics to reduce injuries? Are staff trained in these?
- Is the client changing area clean and stocked with needed items? Is a covered hamper provided for soiled linens and covered trash receptacle for disposable items?
- If in a spa setting, is the shower clean and disinfected?

Other safety protocols will likely be necessary. The information provided here is only general criteria to get you started. Some additional needs to consider may include what items are required prior to opening and before closing for the day. Details that you may consider to be common knowledge, such as accident prevention or client care, are also significant and should not be disregarded; employers should have a safety awareness plan and require all employees to be properly educated on safe practices. A structured plan will lead employees in the establishment to work in a safe manner.

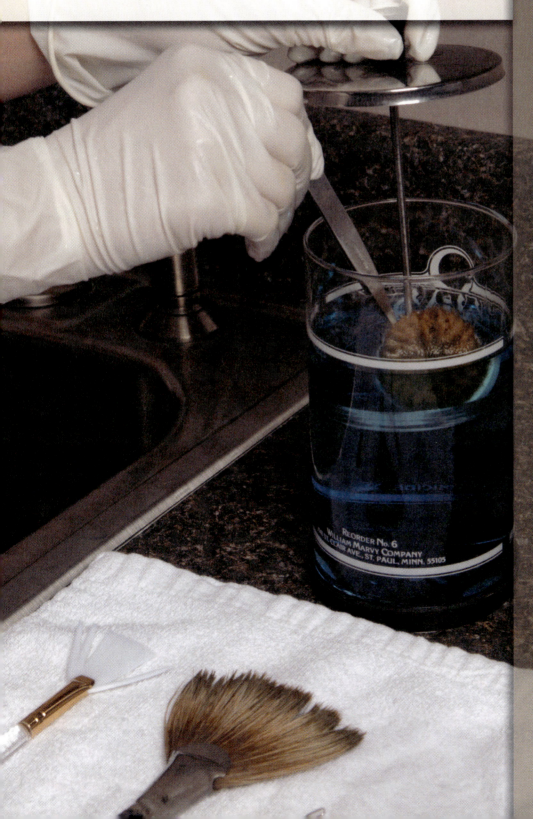

Infection Control

INTRODUCTION

Estheticians routinely have direct, close contact with clients. This chapter will discuss how disease can be spread and the steps we can incorporate into our routine for preventing the spread of disease. The eyes, nose, and mouth are all portals of entrance and exit for transmission of body fluids. For example, staphylococci are commonly found in the flora of the skin but especially in the underarm, groin, and nose areas; the largest concentration in the body is found in the nose. Most of us have tiny microscopic injuries on our hands or along the cuticles which are also portals of entry or exit. Certain strains of herpetic viruses can be transmitted even if there is no active lesion. Herpes may also be moved to another area of the body, which can occur from touching a cold sore followed by touching the genitals. Conjunctivitis, also known as pinkeye, can be triggered by a number of conditions, including simple eye irritation. Standard precautions are published by the Centers for Disease Control and Prevention (CDC) and regulated by the Occupational Safety and Health Administration (OSHA). Following these guidelines will reduce the sharing of diseases and protect our own health and that of our clients. While it may seem intimidating, understanding and following standard precautions makes the process relatively simple.

PATHOGENIC ORGANISMS AND STANDARD PRECAUTIONS

Everyone is constantly being exposed to bacteria, viruses, and other organisms that have the potential to make us ill. These are called pathogenic organisms. Our textbooks detail general classifications of bacteria such as cocci, bacilli, and spirilla (Figure 2–1). Viruses are much smaller than bacteria and function

FIGURE 2-1 Classifications of pathogenic bacteria and the common associated illnesses.

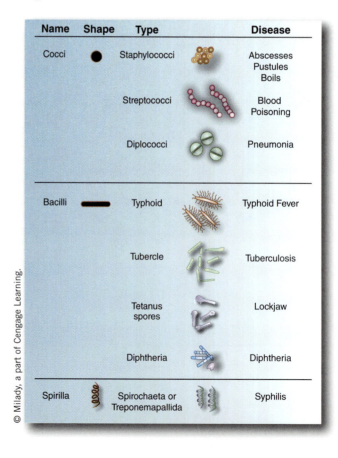

© Milady, a part of Cengage Learning.

Name	Shape	Type		Disease
Cocci	●	Staphylococci		Abscesses Pustules Boils
		Streptococci		Blood Poisoning
		Diplococci		Pneumonia
Bacilli	▬	Typhoid		Typhoid Fever
		Tubercle		Tuberculosis
		Tetanus spores		Lockjaw
		Diphtheria		Diphtheria
Spirilla		Spirochaeta or Treponemapallida		Syphilis

ORGANISM	MODE OF TRANSMISSION
Adenovirus (common cold)	Airborne, direct contact (skin, saliva), fecal-oral, occasionally waterborne, and some surfaces
Herpes simplex 1 virus (oral herpes)	Direct contact with saliva or lesion
Herpes simplex 2 virus (genital herpes)	Direct contact with carrier. Lesions do not have to be present
Influenza virus (common flu)	Airborne, direct and indirect contact
Methicillin-resistant *Staphylococcus aureus* (MRSA)	Direct and indirect contact
Conjunctivitis (eye infection)	Direct (eye-to-hand/hand-to-eye) and indirect contact; dependent on cause
Varicella virus (chicken pox and shingles)	Direct contact or airborne
Mycobacterium tuberculosis (tuberculosis)	Airborne contaminated food or water
Hepatitis type A virus	Contaminated food or water
	Direct and indirect contact
Hepatitis type B, C, or D virus	Contact with blood, bodily fluids, secretions, excretions, mucous membranes, and non-intact skin
Human immunodeficiency virus (precursor of AIDS)	Contact with blood or bodily fluids, secretions, excretions, mucous membranes, and non intact-skin

© Milady, a part of Cengage Learning.

TABLE 2–1 Commonly encountered disease-causing organisms.

differently, but they are equally effective at making us ill. Pathogens may be transmitted by direct or indirect contact with a contaminated surface, object, or person; they may also be airborne, meaning they are transmitted in the air.

While there are many disease-causing organisms, Table 2–1 outlines the most common ones that estheticians will encounter in the course of their work.

PREVENTIVE MEASURES

Pathogenic organisms are spread in a diversity of ways and the esthetician must be prepared to deal with each of them through standard methodology. The Standard Precautions published by the CDC provide this methodology for our use throughout our client care to safeguard ourselves and our clients from pathogens. Standard Precautions instruct us to treat every client and ourselves as if all of us were potential carriers of an infectious organism; this instruction is based on the assumption that all body fluids are infectious. Essential to following this rule are practices of frequent proper hand washing, wearing gloves, and use of appropriate body protection during treatment and clean-up. Employers must provide protective devices such as antiseptic soap, splashguards, masks, eye-flush stations, sharps disposal containers, and labels for all biohazardous materials. Standard Precautions also require workers to wear the necessary personal protective equipment and maintain the work environment in a clean and safe manner. Proper vaccinations are an additional protection method set out in the Standard Precautions. Employers of estheticians in a medical office or clinic must provide the required

FYI

Keep in mind that both forms of Herpes simplex can appear in either the oral or genital region and can be transferred between regions; it can also be spread to the eye (Figure 2–2).

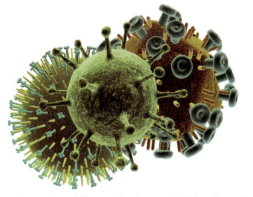

© Sebastian Kaulitzki/www.Shutterstock.com

FIGURE 2–2 Microscopic viruses attack healthy cells.

hepatitis B vaccination. An esthetician working outside a medical office may not be required to have this vaccination but while still at risk of potential exposure may desire to seek the vaccination. Adherence to Standard Precautions includes a close monitoring of some commonly overlooked conditions such as a cold or symptoms that may indicate that a person is carrying a flu virus. With the majority of esthetic treatments occurring on the face, nasal discharge, watery or irritated eyes, coughs, and sneezing are a routine hazard in our industry.

The Standard Precautions guidelines also apply to blood or body fluids, mucous membrane areas, and broken skin, whether or not there is visible evidence of blood. Mucous membranes are found on the face in the region of the eyes, nose, and mouth and on genital areas. The American Red Cross takes this a step farther in its Advisory Council on First Aid and Safety (ACFAS) publication on recommended hand hygiene for the general public. ACFAS guidelines include always washing the hands and using gloves as protective barriers in any situation where there is a risk of non-intact skin or if there is any contact with OPIM (Other Potentially Infectious Material) on non-intact or intact skin ("Hand hygiene for," 2006).

We must remember two key terms and incorporate them into our daily practice. The first is POTENTIAL risk. We may not be able to assess a risk as likely, but if there is a potential for risk, we must take steps to mitigate it. We must also understand Other Potentially Infectious Material (OPIM). In the event that contact occurs with an area where pathogens are known to exist or in cases where a technician may be dealing with non-intact skin, we must take provisions and follow Standard Precautions closely. In some states such as California, used microdermabrasion crystals are considered a biohazard because OPIM could be present in the dead skin that has been exfoliated. Many states have guidelines that clarify the directives from OSHA and the CDC. If directives are specified at the state level, both the state and national standards must be followed. In the event that the state and national standards differ, follow whichever is the stricter of the two. Never assume that because something is not specified at the state level, it does not apply.

Proper hand washing, wearing personal protective equipment such as gloves and safety glasses, and maintaining a clean work environment are all safe practices. Infection control practices will reduce the risk of cross-contamination and prevent the spread of disease. In order to prevent the spread of disease, the CDC has published guidelines for hospital settings, but also requires protective methodologies for nonhospital settings including health care clinics and facilities, schools, and workplace environments. A workplace environment is any place of business, including spas and salons. The hospice division of CDC has listed recommendations for the home environment. All of these recommendations follow

STATE REGULATORY ALERT

If directives are not stated clearly at the state level, then the national standards from OSHA and CDC must be followed. Always compare and follow the stricter of the federal or state regulations to ensure proper compliance.

the same Standard Precautions. Standard Precautions must be adhered to at all times in the workplace and with every treatment.

Vaccinations or immunizations may prevent the risk of contracting some viruses and bacteria. Proper use of immunizations offers superior protection and peace of mind. Currently recommended vaccinations include those for diphtheria, tetanus, pertussis, HPV, hepatitis A, varicella, measles, mumps, rubella, influenza, pneumococcus, and meningococcus (CDC). Annual influenza injections are the best precaution to prevent the spread of the flu. The recommended pneumonia immunizations may prevent colds from developing into this severe and dangerous lung infection. If an employee lacks these vaccinations, the employer is required by OSHA to pay for them.

SAFETY PRACTICES

To help ensure that we are following the Standard Precautions mandated by OSHA, we can create checklists to confirm that we have the equipment and supplies necessary to practice infection control. It is helpful to post these in the dispensary and appointment scheduling area. They should be a part of the employee manual and/or business guide.

Safety Practices Checklist

- Practice proper hand-washing procedures.
- Apply lotions to hands regularly to protect the skin.
- Reschedule any client who appears ill and instruct clients when they schedule to please call in if they are ill and reschedule.
- Refer clients with apparent skin infections to a medical provider.
- Do not work if you are feeling ill or have a communicable disease (this would include a cold).
- Wear protective attire over your street clothes so you don't transmit germs from the workplace to home or vice versa.
- Wear disposable face masks as required by your state or recommended by manufacturers.
- Wear disposable gloves anytime you are performing services where there is an increased risk of cross contamination or contact with body fluids such as:
  - Working around eyes, nose, mouth
  - Working in the underarm, groin, or genital areas
  - Exfoliating the skin (removing layers of epidermal tissue)
  - Performing extraction
  - Any additional time as required by state regulations
- Wear gloves if you have any breaks in the skin of your hands or around nails—keep in mind that even ones that are microscopic in size are still a portal through which pathogens can enter.
- Check fingernails for chips in polish, since chips or small cracks can harbor pathogens.

Keep fingernails short with smooth edges and inspect routinely for signs of skin irritation or infection.

MRSA

Methicillin-resistant *Staphylococcus aureus* (MRSA) is a bacterial infection that is highly resistant to most antibiotics. *Staphylococcus aureus* is a common type of bacteria that normally live on the skin and sometimes in the nasal passages of healthy people. MRSA refers to the specific strain of *Staphylococcus aureus* that does not respond to the common antibiotics used to treat staph infections. This antibiotic resistance results in serious health concerns, longer illnesses, and the potential for death. Be familiar with the common factors of MRSA transmission.

The 5 C's That Contribute to the Spread of MRSA

- Crowding
- Contact with skin
- Compromised skin
- Contaminated items and surfaces
- Cleanliness problems—non-adherence to hand-washing practices

Here are CDC guidelines to prevent contracting a general staphylococcus or MRSA skin infection.

- Practice good hygiene.
- Keep hands clean by washing with soap and water, or alcohol-based sanitizer if the water method of hand washing is not available.
- Keep cuts and scrapes clean and covered with a bandage until healed.
- Avoid contact with other people's wounds or bandages.
- Wear gloves if you must assist with a wound or bandage.
- Avoid sharing personal items such as toothbrush, cosmetics, towels, uniforms, razors, or other items that come into direct skin contact.

Influenza

Influenza is a virus that has cycles of varying intensity. The organism is constantly mutating or changing in its quest for survival. This mutation makes it difficult for scientists, as it quickly becomes resistant to the immunizations developed as prevention. With the increased mobility of the population, the risk of a pandemic has become a great concern. Prevention and adherence to infection-prevention practices are the best deterrents to the spread of influenza. Following safety practices, such as wearing a mask and gloves and adhering closely to hand washing and other infection control practices, can minimize the risk of passing influenza on to others.

Influenza Prevention Checklist

- Get an annual influenza shot.
- Avoid close contact with people who are sick.
- If you are sick, keep your distance from others.
- Stay home—avoid work, errands, school to prevent the spread of the disease.
- Cover your mouth and nose when you cough or sneeze.
- Wash hands often to protect yourself from germs.

- Avoid touching eyes, nose, or mouth, as you may transmit germs to these areas from objects you have touched.
- Practice good health habits—get plenty of rest, exercise, and nutritious food, drink plenty of water, and manage stress.

Conjunctivitis

Conjunctivitis can be described as the (inflammation) or infection of the membrane lining the eyelids (conjunctiva). There are many causes of red or irritated eyes, including bacterial or viral infection and allergic reaction. Irritation of the eye can be uncomfortable for the client; it is therefore important that we employ techniques to minimize this risk in our practice.

Bacterial forms of conjunctivitis are either from cocci or bacilli pathogens. Viruses such as the adenovirus, which causes the common cold, can also lead to conjunctivitis. People who wear contact lenses are more prone to eye irritations that manifest as conjunctivitis. Products entering the eye can cause an allergic or toxic conjunctivitis response.

Conjunctivitis Prevention List

- Wash hands before and after working with each client.
- Reschedule clients who are coming in for any facial treatment if they have symptoms of eye irritation.
- Determine during client consultation if the client has a history of eye infections.
- Use single-use disposable items in the eye area whenever possible.
- Avoid excessive rubbing, tugging, or pressure around the eye.
- Have supplies for flushing the eye immediately available should a client complain of stinging or burning of the eye, and know how to use them.
- Wash your hands before and after touching contact lenses.

GENERAL SAFETY AND SUPPLY CHECKLIST

Safety and supply checklists should be posted in the areas where they will be used. Checklists help us make sure we have the supplies we need to practice safely. Cleaning and disinfecting routines are a critical step to make sure nothing is overlooked. Checklists for cleaning and disinfecting should be created based on how frequently they are performed. Daily, weekly, and monthly or quarterly cleaning and disinfecting routines can ensure an optimum environment. Some clinics have opening and closing routines to ensure that every technician is following the same guidelines and to minimize the unexpected. The items included in each routine will vary depending on the services offered.

Supply checklists help us verify that we have the supplies necessary for safe practice. They are an ongoing reminder to ensure appropriate inventory is maintained. In a large facility, supplies may be inventory controlled; in these cases, a reminder to order a given supply is generated automatically when the stock on hand falls below a certain level. Physical counts are also needed to make sure that the actual count matches the computer-generated figures.

Supply Checklist

- Adequate cleaning and disinfecting supplies as approved by your state
- EPA-registered hospital disinfectant
- Safety glasses to wear when mixing disinfectants
- Disposable single-use gloves in appropriate sizes
- Cleaning gloves
- Closed storage receptacle for clean linens
- Closed storage receptacle for dirty and biohazardous linens
- Cleaning tools: mop, broom, vacuum, disposable towels, and scrub brushes
- Cleaning agents and detergents for laundry, sink, hands, floors, and walls
- Paper supplies: towels, tissues, toilet paper
- First-aid kit with adequate supplies
- Closed storage receptacle for waste or general trash
- Closed storage receptacle for biohazardous waste
- Receptacles for contaminated sharps

ASEPSIS

Asepsis is the state of being free from disease-causing contaminants. The term also often refers to those practices used to promote or induce asepsis in a specific area in an effort to prevent infection. A contaminated environment is a perfect incubator for microorganisms. An aseptic—literally, "against septic"—environment is the opposite. An aseptic situation is one that does not provide for the growth of microorganisms. When performing services or treatments for clients, we want to have as aseptic an environment as possible. There are five keys to asepsis:

1. Know what has been cleaned and is disinfected.
2. Know what is contaminated.
3. Know what is sterile.
4. Keep clean, contaminated, and sterile items separated.
5. Resolve contamination immediately by cleaning and then disinfecting, or cleaning and then sterilizing.

Knowledge of asepsis is as useful in pre- and post-service preparation as it is in arranging and maintaining the dispensary. Key ways to ensure asepsis include not placing contaminated treatment items randomly over the work area, immediately placing disposables (single-use items) into a proper waste receptacle and sharps into a sharps container, and dividing the work area setup into zones for disinfected, sterile, and used non-disposable (multi-use) items.

HAND CLEANSING AND CARE

According to the CDC, proper hand washing is the single most important factor in preventing the spread of infection or disease. Proper hand washing should be completed using liquid soap or antibacterial cleanser, running water, and a nail brush to clean the sides and under the nail plate. Alcohol-based, waterless hand cleansers are not recommended when the hands are visibly dirty or contaminated with proteinaceous materials. Otherwise, alcohol-based, waterless hand cleansers have been found to be just as effective at reducing the number of pathogens on the skin as hand washing (CDC). When washing the hands, the water used should be warm, not cold or hot. Hot water opens the pores of the skin, leaving it vulnerable to microorganisms, and cold water may not readily dissolve oils. Rinse the hands thoroughly and blot away excess water; never aggressively rub the hands dry. Care should be taken to avoid dry, irritated, or chapped hands; routine use of lotions to moisturize the skin is beneficial. Care should be taken that the lotion selected will not compromise the quality of protective gloves.

Proper hand washing must be done for various reasons. Provided for you is a list of times you should practice hand washing.

- Wash hands often, including upon arrival at work and before and after every client.
- Some states require hand washing prior to the application of gloves.
- After the removal of gloves
- After contact with any potentially contaminated surface or object
- After working in common areas
- Between clients with whom you have had direct contact
- Before and after eating
- After using the restroom
- Any time hands are visibly soiled or after sneezing, coughing, or blowing your nose
- Before leaving work
- Whenever common sense indicates proper hand washing is warranted

Hand-Washing Protocol

For hand washing to be effective, it must be completed in the listed order and by following each step.

- Hand washing should be done with warm running water and take a minimum of 20 seconds.
- First, wet your hands with warm running water.
- Apply a small, yet sufficient, amount of liquid soap (either antimicrobial or plain) and thoroughly distribute over hands, cuticles, and fingernails (Figure 2–3).
- Vigorously rub together all surfaces of lathered hands for 20 seconds (Figure 2–4).
  - Inter-digitally (between the fingers)
  - Don't forget those thumbs!
  - Wrists
  - Nail beds
  - Beneath fingernails using a nail brush
  - Palms of hands
- Pump soap on a clean, disinfected nail brush nails horizontally and vertically and brush along nail folds of fingernails. (Figure 2–5).
- Thoroughly rinse your hands (from the top of the wrist down to the fingertips) under warm running water to remove residual soap (Figure 2–6).

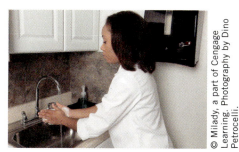

FIGURE 2–3 Wet your hands, apply soap (liquid antimicrobial or plain) and distribute thoroughly.

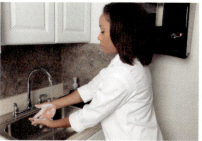

FIGURE 2–4 Vigorously rub all hand surfaces for 20 seconds paying special attention to area surrounding and underneath fingernails, between the fingers and the palms.

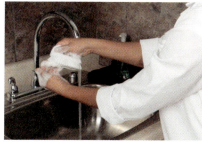

FIGURE 2–5 Pump soap on a clean, disinfected nail brush nails horizontally and vertically and brush along nail folds of fingernails.

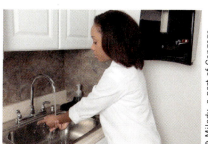

FIGURE 2–6 Thoroughly rinse from the wrists toward the fingertips using warm running water.

© Milady, a part of Cengage Learning. Photography by Dino Petrocelli.

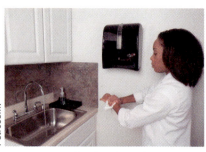

FIGURE 2–7 Pat dry with a disposable paper towel.

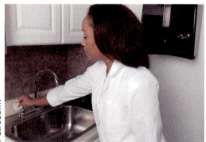

FIGURE 2–8 Avoid recontamination by using a disposable paper towel to turn off the water.

- Blot or pat—do not rub—the hands dry with a disposable paper towel (Figure 2–7).
- Avoid recontamination. Use a foot control or the paper towel to turn off the water (Figure 2–8). Do not touch the faucet with your hand.
- As an optional step, apply hand lotion as needed.

Hand Care

The hands are an important tool for an esthetician, so it is important to care for them. To prevent breaking the client's skin when performing esthetic services, the free edge of the fingernail should be no longer than 1/8 inch. When viewing your hands from the palm side, the nails should not be visible over the tips of the fingers. Nail enhancements must be kept short and meticulously maintained to prevent the growth of pathogens in cracks or if there is lifting. An esthetician wearing enhancements should wear gloves when performing services as a prevention protocol. Improper application and maintenance of nail enhancements can traumatize cuticles or adjacent skin, leaving minute wounds. To reduce the risk of irritation or infection, never cut the cuticle. Application of moisturizing products can prevent dry and chapped skin on the hands. Visible or invisible breaks (microtrauma) in the skin or cuticles result from chapped or dry skin; any break in the skin allows a point of entry for bacteria or viruses.

Glove Selection

Gloves should be selected based on fit, the type of service being offered, and the products to be used while wearing the gloves (Figure 2–9). Incorrect selection or identification of the glove being used could lead to a client skin reaction or to the technician not having the protection they need. Purchasing different colors of gloves for each of the different sizes or based on the type of glove material can simplify and facilitate the correct selection of the glove.

Latex gloves have become less popular due to an increase in clients/technicians with latex allergies or sensitivities. If technicians are using products with oil in them, the oil immediately compromises the latex glove barrier protection even though this will not be visually detectable.

Nitrile gloves are popular with those performing permanent makeup services, but if they fit poorly their tactile surface makes them less desirable for skin care, as they can drag on the skin. Nitrile gloves are very resistant to many chemicals and oil-based products but these gloves are not as flexible and have less stretch than some other types.

Vinyl or new polyvinyl chloride (PVC) blends offer a combination of slip and grip. These PVC blends are more elastic and have good tactile sensitivity. Vinyl gloves have good puncture resistance and are resistant

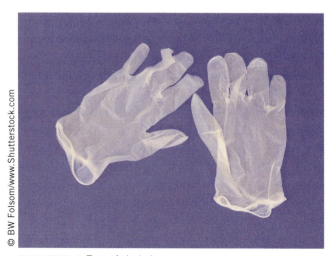

FIGURE 2–9 Type of vinyl gloves.

to oxidation, many acids, alkalis, fats, and alcohols. The vinyl and PVC-blend gloves do not have resistance to organic solvents.

Glove manufacturers will be able to offer assistance in choosing the best glove for the treatments and products you use. The manufacturer can provide you with glove testing results, which include suggested chemical use and levels of stress. A reference chart for glove materials and selection for use is found in the *Milady Standard Esthetics: Advanced* textbook.

It is also important to keep in mind that, while protective, the constant use of gloves may lead to an irritant dermatitis condition. Some people develop irritation from the glove itself, from glove powders, from the increased perspiration of their hands, or even from soap residue left from hand washing. Irritant dermatitis conditions can appear as severely chapped skin and for some may develop into an allergic dermatitis. Irritation can be prevented with the use of thin cotton gloves available to be worn as liners under gloves.

BARRIER FILM

Barrier film is an inexpensive product readily available through medical supply firms that can be a great preventive measure for the esthetician (Figure 2–10). This product is available in rolls of clear or blue film from medical supply distributors and is a dense, pliable plastic with perforated squares that can be easily torn off and applied to equipment or products, providing an efficient method of avoiding cross-contamination. Dentists and permanent makeup technicians use barrier films routinely on equipment they will be touching with a potentially contaminated hand. Estheticians can use barrier film on magnifying lamps, switches, or containers that will need to be handled during a treatment (Figure 2–11). Using barrier films can speed up the cleaning and disinfection process and reduce the chance of labeling being removed due to repeated exposure to disinfectants or cleaning agents. On a complex object such as a magnifying lamp, which has no flat surface that can be easily wiped down, using barrier film on the areas to be handled reduces the risk of cross-contamination. It is also practical for use on equipment components that are not easily removed for disinfection. Contact your equipment manufacturer before applying barrier film to digital readout touch screens to make sure that they are compatible.

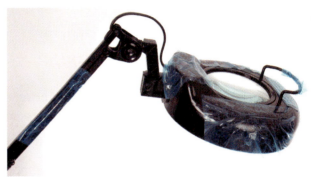

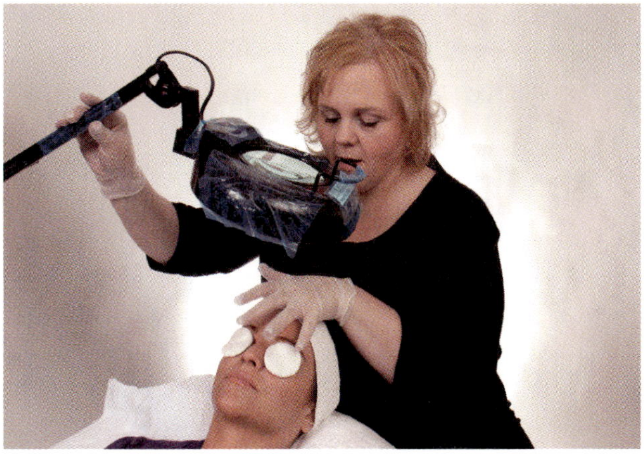

FIGURE 2-10 Barrier film can be purchased in rolls for custom sizing.

© Milady, a part of Cengage Learning. Photography by Visual Recollections.

FIGURE 2-11 Barrier film placed on a mag lamp.

© Milady, a part of Cengage Learning. Photography by Visual Recollections.

DECONTAMINATION

Decontamination of our equipment, tools, and work environment is an integral part of a safe esthetics practice. There are three levels of decontamination. The lowest level is cleaning, which removes a majority of pathogens but does not guarantee complete pathogen elimination. Disinfection kills all microorganisms but does not kill spores. Only sterilization, the highest level of decontamination, has the ability to kill spores, which are resistant to heat, drying, and the action of disinfectants.

Cleaning alone is not adequate for the decontamination of esthetic tools or implements or work surfaces. They are mostly practiced for the general maintenance of the workplace environment. State regulatory agencies require estheticians to clean and then disinfect tools, implements, and work surfaces.

Cleaning

Cleaning is the first step in the disinfection or sterilization process. Before an item can be disinfected or sterilized, it must be properly cleaned. Proper cleaning of an item begins with removal of all soil, debris, or foreign material from the implement or equipment. The item must then be properly washed with warm water and a detergent designed for removal of all dirt and oils. Completion of the cleaning process must be followed by a thorough rinsing and proper drying process.

Steps for Cleaning and Disinfection

- Remove any gross debris, including hair, wax, etc.
- Scrub under running water to remove any remaining debris.
- Rinse and blot to remove excess moisture.
- Completely immerse tools and implements in disinfecting solution following manufacturer guidelines.
- Understand and follow the directions for required contact time to be effective against pathogens.
- Rinse afterward to remove the disinfecting agent from the implement.
- Dry thoroughly before storing in a clean and closed container.

Disinfection

There are multiple types of disinfectants available, and they should be selected for use based on what is being disinfected. All disinfectants are pesticides so they must be registered with the Environmental Protection Agency (EPA) and should have an EPA registration number clearly listed on the label. All instruments coming into contact with clients must be properly disinfected prior to use. This process must be completed in advance and cannot be hurried in any situation.

Disinfection of Items

Esthetic items that must be disinfected include any object that has the potential to be exposed to blood and body fluids, OPIM, or contaminated items; and all items that come in contact with non-intact unbroken skin. These may be divided into categories of critical, semi-critical, and noncritical items.

Examples of critical items include anything sharp, comedone extractors, tweezers, or any other items that come into contact with non-intact skin.

FYI

Complete decontamination of an implement or tool cannot be achieved with disinfection or sterilization alone. You must first clean the item and then follow up with the required method of decontamination. Any item that has not been properly cleaned first does not produce a decontaminated result.

Semi-critical items are those that do not penetrate the body but may be exposed to OPIM or other contaminated items. Examples of semi-critical items are work surfaces, equipment, and other inanimate objects that do not penetrate any surface of the body. Semi-critical items will potentially be exposed to blood, body fluids, OPIM, or other contamination. Sterilization is not feasible for these items, so the use of barrier protection, cleaning, and disinfecting are essential. We may use an intermediate-level disinfectant that kills vegetative microorganisms, tuberculosis, fungi, and small viruses. This will not kill bacterial spores. Follow manufacturers' directions for use and replacement of this disinfectant.

The third category is noncritical items, which only come in contact with unbroken skin or indirect contact with the client. Floors, walls, and furnishings are examples of noncritical items. They can be cleaned using a low-level disinfectant, a type of disinfectant that cannot be relied on to kill spores, tuberculosis, fungi, or viruses.

Knowledge of the three categories of items and disinfectants may be used for guidance in the process of selecting a disinfectant.

Selecting a Disinfectant

Here is a checklist of factors for selection and purchase of a disinfectant:

- Level of disinfection required
- Limitations of the product
- How tools and equipment should be cleaned before exposing them to the disinfectant
- Whether or not the disinfectant is user-friendly
- Special preparations needed to prepare tools or equipment for the disinfection process
- Potential toxicity
- Specific instructions explaining how to avoid toxic conditions or reactions during use
- Storage conditions
- Does the disinfectant leave any residue on tools or equipment that could be potentially toxic to clients or staff?
- Are there potential physical hazards such as fire or explosion?
- Can heat or environmental conditions cause chemical changes to the disinfectant?

Sterilization

Sterilization is the decontamination process that will kill all living organisms, including spores. Most commonly, sterilization is referred to as heat sterilization; this is the process of exposing cleaned implements or tools to specified temperatures at high pressure for a specific period of time. This method involves the use of an autoclave, which generates pressurized steam. The manufacturer of this type of equipment must submit to the FDA, prior to marketing, technical data demonstrating that sterilization has occurred and is maintainable once the procedure is over. Steam, dry heat, and unsaturated chemical vapor are the only methodologies currently approved by the FDA as sterilization methods. In the

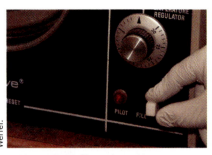

FIGURE 2–12 Properly package implements prior to autoclaving.

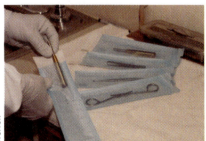

FIGURE 2–13 Follow instructions from the manufacturer to properly load an autoclave.

medi-spa and esthetic industry, use of an autoclave on all critical items is the preferred method (Figure 2–12).

FDA requirements are followed to ensure that proper sterilization occurs. A temperature gauge on the outside of the autoclave is monitored to make sure the appropriate temperature and pressure are maintained within the unit to kill all organisms (Figure 2–13). The length or duration of the cycle varies with the unit model and with whether a load is the first of the morning, a cold start, or one later in the day, after the unit has been run repeatedly and retains heat from previous cycles. The high pressure is necessary to raise the temperature of the water above the boiling point, and an external pressure gauge indicates the level of pressure and the safe operating range. A timer on the unit is used to ensure that the correct pressure and temperature are maintained long enough to destroy all living organisms. This process commonly involves maintaining a temperature of 274°F for 15 minutes.

Another helpful and necessary tool is small integrators, available from medical supply firms. These integrators are run with each load to demonstrate sterilization. Integrators respond to heat, pressure, and duration to show that a cycle is complete. They do not prove sterilization, however; they only show that a sterilization unit is operating properly.

Anyone using an autoclave should use routine biological monitoring, also called spore testing. This testing, commonly performed once a month, is used to ensure that the unit is actually sterilizing items. Special packets available from testing providers have two pockets in the envelope. One side contains a testing strip and the other side a control strip. Each of these strips is in its own little packet. The testing strip, still in its packet, is placed in the autoclave and run through a normal load cycle. Then it is placed back into the envelope and sent to the testing firm, which will return a report explaining whether the device is sterilizing effectively and indicating if there is a problem.

Following the completion of a sterilization cycle, the autoclave must either be "vented" or processed through a drying cycle. This allows moisture to escape from the unit rather than being absorbed into the packaging materials.

Sterilization of Implements

Any implement to be sterilized must go through a cleaning process prior to sterilization. After the tool is clean and dry, it is usually then placed in a paper or plastic sleeve. The sleeve offers proper storage and maintains sterility following the process. This sleeve or pouch is commonly paper on one side and plastic on the other so that the item is clearly visible. One end of the pouch will be open so that the item can be slid into it, then the top folded down and sealed into place. The pouch should not be overfilled, and as much air as possible should be removed prior to sealing. Leave about 1 inch of space between the contents and the sealed edges.

After sterilization check the packaging to ensure it has not become saturated with moisture, which could compromise the barrier of the packaging and thus the sterility of the item. If this has occurred, the item will need to be repackaged and reprocessed. All properly sterilized items should remain in the package and be placed in a designated clean, dry storage area. Packages may also be labeled

> **CAUTION**
>
> Autoclaves are units that employ heat, steam, and pressure to eliminate all life forms. It is important that anyone operating one be trained in its use and follow all manufacturer guidelines.

with the date of the sterilization process so that items may be used on a timely basis.

Working with Sharps

It is critical to practice skills of safe use when working with any instrument termed as a "sharp." The definition of a sharp is any object with a point or sharp edge that could penetrate, cut, or otherwise break the skin. Estheticians use tweezers, eyebrow scissors, comedone extractors, lancets (in states where they are allowed), and other sharp devices. Any sharp implement must either be single-use and disposed of after use, or processed through disinfection or autoclaving. Sharps that are to be disposed of must be placed in a designated sharps container that meets OSHA and CDC guidelines (Figure 2–14). It is recommended not to overfill a sharps container (usually use only up to 2/3 of its capacity). Overfilling a sharps container may lead to an inadvertent stick by someone else later on who is handling the container. Gloves, cotton swabs, or towels used to clean up blood or fluids should be put in a plastic bag, which is then tied and thrown into the garbage. Your locality may require this type of item to be double bagged and labeled with biohazard warning.

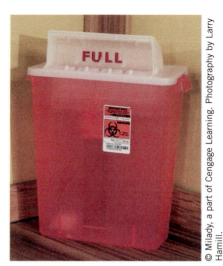

FIGURE 2-14 Example of a sharps container meeting OSHA and CDC guidelines.

© Milady, a part of Cengage Learning. Photography by Larry Hamill.

OSHA also has specific guidelines for the handling of sharp objects. If a sharp such as a lancet is dropped, it should not be picked up with the fingers. Instead, tweezers, forceps, or another device should be used to retrieve it to reduce the risk of accidental sticks. Sharp items should never be recapped, bent, or broken from their base.

Another risk within the clinic is broken glass. Glass is considered a sharp and should be cleaned up using utmost caution. Large pieces can be collected using tweezers, forceps, or tongs. Small pieces should be swept into a dustbin and disposed of. They should not be picked up bare-handed or even with gloved fingers, as this barrier could be easily cut by sharp fragments.

It is important to always be aware that proper decontamination is your responsibility. Take all measures necessary to prevent the spread of infection or disease before and after every client and every treatment. Never allow yourself to feel that something may be skipped or shortened due to time constraints. Careful advance planning allows ample time for being prepared to offer the ultimate treatments.

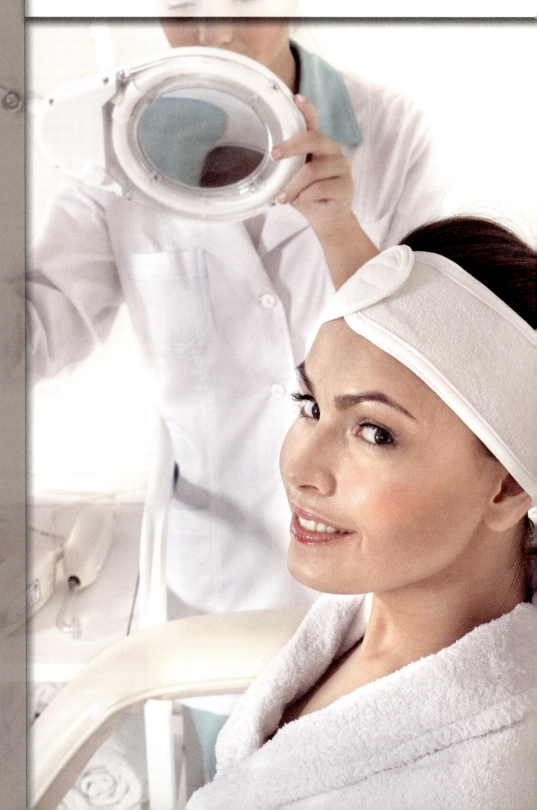

Workplace Safety

INTRODUCTION

A safe working environment is not only beneficial to us and our clients; it is also requirement of federal and state regulations. The federal agencies that mandate some of these regulations are OSHA (Occupational Safety and Health Administration), which is under the Department of Labor; the CDC (Centers for Disease Control), which is under the Department of Health and Human Services; and NIOSH (National Institute for Occupational Safety and Health), which is operated under the CDC. Other regulations are issued by local organizations, including individual state licensing boards and departments of health. Diligent practice of workplace safety allows us to offer our services while minimizing risk of injury or accident to both ourselves and our clients (Figure 3–1). It is critical to practice accident prevention with preparedness, careful planning, and close attention to details. Becoming knowledgeable about federal and local standards, common accident causes, prevention techniques, and risk management will help an esthetician to develop more effective safety practices.

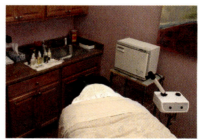

FIGURE 3–1 A safely prepared treatment room.

FEDERAL STANDARDS

OSHA, the CDC, and NIOSH are all federal agencies that offer protection to workers from on-the-job harm. Specifically, OSHA's mission is to prevent work-related injuries, illnesses, and occupational fatalities by issuing and enforcing standards for workplace safety and health. The goal of the CDC is to look for ways to protect everyone from the spread of disease. The NIOSH agency is responsible for conducting research and making recommendations for the prevention of work-related injury and illness.

OSHA

OSHA was created within the U.S. Department of Labor to encourage both employers and employees to implement safer work and health practices to reduce on-the-job hazards. This includes responsibility for the development and implementation of training programs to increase the competency of health and safety personnel. Simply stated, OSHA has the job of creating guidelines to keep workers safe in their work environments. Originally, the guidelines were called the Safety Bill of Rights and the Worker's Right to Know Act; each set of guidelines was developed so that workers would know and recognize hazardous chemicals and conditions in the workplace. Both sets of guidelines were also designed to minimize accidents or situations that could affect the health of the worker. Many states have chosen to administer the OSHA program as it is; others have adapted the regulations and created standards that are at least as strict as the federal regulations. All states must at a minimum follow the OSHA-prescribed standards. "Standard of care" may be explained as the watchfulness, attention, caution, and prudence a reasonable person would exercise within his or her profession. Failure to meet the standard of care is considered negligence. All employees should take the time to become knowledgeable of the expected standards of care for their area of industry.

Hazards Communication Standard

An additional aspect of OSHA standards is the application of the Hazards Communication Standard. This standard says that all employees have the right to know about the chemicals they work with and the hazards associated with those chemicals. In the esthetics industry, this would include cleaning agents, skin-care treatment products, and any other chemicals that may cause problems for the technician. It is important to always remember that chemicals may be hazardous even if they are commonly used and may not appear dangerous.

All facilities that have hazardous chemicals must have a written plan describing how the Hazards Communication Standard will be implemented in that facility. This plan must indicate:

- Chemicals present in the clinic.
- Who is responsible for the aspects of the program in the clinic.
- Where written materials on the chemicals are available to employees.
- How the requirements for this and other forms of warning, MSDS sheets, and employee information are met within the facility.

While we think of OSHA as being just for industry and construction or larger businesses, it applies to all businesses with more than 10 employees. OSHA has determined that the leaseholder of a facility that rents work areas becomes in this case the "host" employer, and all within that facility must follow OSHA guidelines. Even for those who are exempt from the rule, following these safety and protection guidelines is essential for operating a safe clinic environment.

OSHA and the CDC are closely tied together, with some overlap. While OSHA focuses on worker and workplace safety, the CDC focuses on preventing the spread of disease. OSHA is focused more on employees, while the CDC covers everyone. In the case of an accident resulting in injury, both organizations could be involved. OSHA may investigate for safety practices, examining how the accident could have been prevented and potential workplace risks to the employee. The CDC could be involved in any situation in which a contagious outbreak or unknown source of infection were a concern.

CDC and the Bloodborne Pathogens Standard

The Centers for Disease Control developed the Bloodborne Pathogens standard to minimize the transmission of HIV and hepatitis B infections among health care workers. This covers all employees who can be "reasonably anticipated" to come into contact, through the course of performing their duties, with blood and other potentially infectious materials (OPIM). This standard has been expanded to create guidelines for non–health care settings and includes any situation where the risk of bloodborne pathogen transmission is present.

FYI

The CDC developed the guidelines for the Bloodborne Pathogens standard, but because the CDC has no regulatory authority, it offered the recommendations to OSHA. OSHA then turned the Bloodborne Pathogens standard into a rule that was subsequently passed into law.

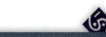

STATE REGULATORY ALERT

Many states offer free on-line OSHA training programs so that employers and employees can be familiar with the ways to control risks. Check with your licensing agency or local OSHA representatives.

Important components of the Bloodborne Pathogens standard include reducing risk or limiting exposure, identifying possible modes of transmission, and complying with regulations.

REDUCING RISK

The most common method of reducing of risk transmission of bloodborne pathogens is practicing standard precautions and correct use of personal protective equipment (PPE). PPE items are used for the protection of the skin, face, and eyes; PPE commonly used by an esthetician will include gloves, masks, or facial shield techniques and proper clothing (Figure 3–2).

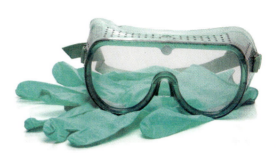

FIGURE 3-2 Personal protection equipment includes items for protection of the skin and eyes.

© Rob Byron/www.Shutterstock.com

Modes of Transmission

Bloodborne pathogens such as HBV and human immunodeficiency virus (HIV) can be transmitted through contact with infected human blood and other potentially infectious bodily fluids, mucous membranes, and non-intact skin.

It is important to know the ways that exposure and transmission are most likely to occur in your particular situation. Some instances include providing first aid to a client in the waxing room, handling contaminated laundry, or cleaning up blood from any clinic area or bathroom accident.

Unbroken skin forms an impervious barrier against bloodborne pathogens, but once that barrier breaks down, infected blood can enter your system in many ways. Infections can be transmitted directly through open sores, cuts, abrasions, acne, or any other type of damaged or broken skin such as sunburn or blisters. Bloodborne pathogens may also be transmitted through the mucous membranes of the eyes, nose, mouth, and genital areas. It is important to understand that it can take up to three or more days for broken skin to heal enough to form an intact barrier once more.

Because of their close contact with clients, technicians may find themselves in any number of potentially infection-transmitting situations. A splash of contaminated blood to the eye, nose, or mouth, for example, could result in bloodborne pathogen transmission. During extraction, a lesion could rupture and splatter a technician on the face or in the eye if he or she were not using protective

FYI

Gloves should be selected based on possible allergic reaction and the protection offered by the glove. Some key factors when choosing gloves are the duration of the treatment, the type of treatment, what products the gloves will be exposed to, client and technician sensitivities, and personal preferences. Glove integrity can be affected by certain ingredients in lotions, especially petroleum, and improperly dried hands.

equipment such as safety glasses or a magnifying loupe. A client with nasal discharge is frequently the culprit for transmitting infections and illnesses.

Compliance Program

Following OSHA guidelines is a multistep process. You must maintain proper documentation of your efforts and the results of compliance. The written document itself and the successful implementation of the program are both important. An effective program is based on four cornerstones: involvement by management and employees, an analysis of the worksite, preventing and controlling hazards and safety, and health training.

Owners and managers must set an example and then require all employees and independent contractors to take an active role in the creation and implementation of the plan. There must be guidelines for accountability on the part of both management and staff. OSHA requires that management clearly establish a workplace health and safety policy, that they create a specific goal and objective for the program, and that they be actively involved in implementation.

An example of a goal and implementation might be to reduce the number of workplace accidents or to implement steps to reduce hazards. In a spa setting, a goal may be to prevent falls from slippery floors. The reduction of hazard could be worded as follows: "Immediately upon recognition by any employee, steps are to be implemented to clean and wipe up any liquids or products as to prevent slips on wet floors." You could even have small signs posted in areas where spills may occur, requesting that clients inform an employee if they see any spills on the floor.

Once this commitment is made, the next step in creating a safe workplace will be a complete analysis of it. Any uncertainties or confusion relating to your specific work environment may be researched on the Internet at www.osha.gov.

The worksite analysis is something each team member should be involved in. This is not a one-time project but an ongoing undertaking that will need to be reviewed and updated any time there is an accident, or at least annually. If new equipment or products are purchased, they should be evaluated to identify any potential hazards and establish steps to control or minimize risk. Every facility should be evaluated for safety; this will determine for each area what risks exist and what actions must be taken to eliminate or control them.

In addition to the facility evaluation, job tasks should be analyzed for hazards. A good example is the mixing of concentrated disinfectant chemicals, which presents the risk of splash and injury to the eye or a spill onto exposed skin. Risks can be reduced by using protective eyewear and gloves and providing training in the proper mixing of the chemicals. It should be a requirement that all employees be informed of safe practices and individual understanding is documented. One method of doing may be to require employee signatures following completion of specific training, and to document their understanding.

Employees cannot follow safety guidelines if they are uninformed or do not understand them. Offering education to all new employees and refresher information for existing employees is a critical part of the safety program. The esthetician needs training, often hands-on training, to ensure that every employee understands the techniques that lead to safety and hazard control. Videos are great teaching tools, but they don't offer feedback and suggestions for improving technique.

When planning safety training events, keep in mind that people remember:

- 10% of what they read
- 20% of what they hear
- 30% of what they see
- 50% of what they see and hear
- 70% of what they say
- 90% of what they see and do concurrently when performing a skill or doing homework, papers, or assignments

Often, estheticians work in their treatment rooms alone. As licensed professionals, estheticians must be proactive in learning the hazards of their work areas and diligent in working to prevent or control those hazards. They must seek out both the education and the training necessary to use chemicals and equipment safely. They must also maintain documentation of all safety training for employees, including specific techniques or equipment.

Since this profession is in contact with the general public, it is important to elicit client support in following safety guidelines. This will be reflected in the proper use of client history forms and providing accurate information so that we can offer them the best, safest treatments. Failure to provide a client with a proper interview and clear communication could have disastrous results.

Compliance Checklist

Based on the information from the OSHA Web site, here is a checklist of considerations when applying the four key guidelines of the compliance program. These are provided as a guide and may need to be modified to fit the needs of each business.

1. Create clear safety and health policies and post them so they are readily available to clients and staff.
2. Complete a facility inspection and create a safety checklist for each area.
3. Review the checklist to make sure it is current and being followed.
4. Review the work area safety inspection routinely to detect new hazards and implement changes as needed.
5. Encourage clients to participate in health and safety practices.
6. Accident or health trends should be evaluated and steps taken to reduce or control the triggering factors.
7. Create written safety practices for dealing with hazardous chemicals or situations where some risk is involved.
8. Educate and train all staff on identifying and preventing potential risks or hazards, and the safety procedures necessary to mitigate them.
9. Create a schedule for equipment and facility maintenance tasks to ensure safe operations.
10. Create a plan to deal with potential emergencies, including fire- and weather-related issues.
11. Create a plan to deal with emergencies where first aid assistance may be needed.

12. Create a plan for emergencies that require additional support from a nearby physician or emergency care provider.
13. Document every injury or accident that requires more than basic first aid.

Evaluate each documented injury for steps that can be implemented to prevent its reoccurrence.

Compliance Recordkeeping

OSHA has created special forms that they recommend be used to facilitate the tracking of injuries and illnesses. These forms are available for download on their Web site, www.osha.gov. However, according to OSHA's Standard Industrial Classification (SIC) codes, Beauty Salons SIC 723, Barber Shops SIC 724, and Miscellaneous Personal Services SIC 738 fall under the "partially exempt facilities" category. Based on this classification system, esthetic clinics and day spas would be in this partially exempt category.

Partially exempt facilities are not required to keep OSHA injury and illness records for, unless asked to do so in writing by OSHA, the Bureau of Labor Statistics (BLS), or a state agency operating under the authority of OSHA, or the BLS (Occupational Safety and Health Administration, 2001). All employers, including those partially exempted by reason of company size or industry classification, must report to OSHA any workplace incident that results in a fatality or the hospitalization of three or more employees (Figure 3–3).

While OSHA may not require documentation from your establishment, keeping track of accidents or injuries can be invaluable if they result in litigation. Check with your insurance provider for the preferred forms and reporting methods. If no generic forms are available, the one on the next page will provide a guide for the important information to include. You cannot predict when a small accident could develop into something more significant than it originally appears and later lead to litigation. Keep reporting accurate, thorough, and to the facts.

NIOSH

The National Institute for Occupational Safety and Health (or NIOSH) is the United States federal agency responsible for conducting research and making recommendations for the prevention of work-related injury and illness. NIOSH is part of the Centers for Disease Control and Prevention (CDC) within the U.S. Department of Health and Human Services. NIOSH is not a regulatory agency but instead issues health standards. The NIOSH organization offers a broad range of information that can be beneficial if you have unanswered questions concerning workplace safety. Some of the general topic areas concerning workplace safety and health include industries and occupations, hazards and exposures, diseases and injuries, safety and prevention, chemicals, and emergency preparedness and response. This would be an excellent place to look for information in the event you encounter a unique situation or if a client has a condition that is not commonly encountered by an esthetician.

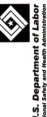

U.S. Department of Labor
Occupational Safety and Health Administration

OSHA's Form 301
Injury and Illness Incident Report

Form approved OMB no. 1218-0176

Attention: This form contains information relating to employee health and must be used in a manner that protects the confidentiality of employees to the extent possible while the information is being used for occupational safety and health purposes.

This *Injury and Illness Incident Report* is one of the first forms you must fill out when a recordable work-related injury or illness has occurred. Together with the *Log of Work-Related Injuries and Illnesses* and the accompanying *Summary*, these forms help the employer and OSHA develop a picture of the extent and severity of work-related incidents.

Within 7 calendar days after you receive information that a recordable work-related injury or illness has occurred, you must fill out this form or an equivalent. Some state workers' compensation, insurance, or other reports may be acceptable substitutes. To be considered an equivalent form, any substitute must contain all the information asked for on this form.

According to Public Law 91-596 and 29 CFR 1904, OSHA's recordkeeping rule, you must keep this form on file for 5 years following the year to which it pertains.

If you need additional copies of this form, you may photocopy and use as many as you need.

Information about the employee

1) Full name _____

2) Street _____
City _____ State _____ ZIP _____

3) Date of birth ___/___/___

4) Date hired ___/___/___

5) ☐ Male
☐ Female

Information about the physician or other health care professional

6) Name of physician or other health care professional _____

7) If treatment was given away from the worksite, where was it given?
Facility _____
Street _____
City _____ State _____ ZIP _____

8) Was employee treated in an emergency room?
☐ Yes
☐ No

9) Was employee hospitalized overnight as an in-patient?
☐ Yes
☐ No

Completed by _____

Title _____

Phone (___) ___ - ___   Date ___/___/___

Information about the case

10) Case number from the *Log* _____ (Transfer the case number from the Log after you record the case.)

11) Date of injury or illness ___/___/___

12) Time employee began work _____ AM / PM

13) Time of event _____ AM / PM ☐ Check if time cannot be determined

14) **What was the employee doing just before the incident occurred?** Describe the activity, as well as the tools, equipment, or material the employee was using. Be specific. *Examples:* "climbing a ladder while carrying roofing materials"; "spraying chlorine from hand sprayer"; "daily computer key-entry."

15) **What happened?** Tell us how the injury occurred. *Examples:* "When ladder slipped on wet floor, worker fell 20 feet"; "Worker was sprayed with chlorine when gasket broke during replacement"; "Worker developed soreness in wrist over time."

16) **What was the injury or illness?** Tell us the part of the body that was affected and how it was affected; be more specific than "hurt," "pain," or sore." *Examples:* "strained back"; "chemical burn, hand"; "carpal tunnel syndrome."

17) **What object or substance directly harmed the employee?** *Examples:* "concrete floor"; "chlorine"; "radial arm saw." *If this question does not apply to the incident, leave it blank.*

18) **If the employee died, when did death occur?** Date of death ___/___/___

Public reporting burden for this collection of information is estimated to average 22 minutes per response, including time for reviewing instructions, searching existing data sources, gathering and maintaining the data needed, and completing and reviewing the collection of information. Persons are not required to respond to the collection of information unless it displays a current valid OMB control number. If you have any comments about this estimate or any other aspects of this data collection, including suggestions for reducing this burden, contact: US Department of Labor, OSHA Office of Statistics, Room N-3644, 200 Constitution Avenue, NW, Washington, DC 20210. Do not send the completed forms to this office.

FIGURE 3-3 OSHA Incident Report Form.

SAFETY PLANNING

A comprehensive general safety checklist is provided in Chapter 1. Create an organized filing system in the clinic or workplace so that needed information can be quickly and easily located. Continue to reevaluate in consideration of any new or additional hazards or changes in practices. Check with your state regulatory agency or state division of OSHA for suggested safety or self-inspection checklists.

Off-Site Treatments

If an esthetician is doing treatments outside a facility, such as in a client's home or on location, then additional considerations should be made. Be sure to tour the environment and consider factors that will impact your service. This will allow you to be properly prepared to perform a quality treatment.

Off-Site Factors to Consider:

- Will you be able to safely transport and set up all equipment and supplies in the location without personal injury?
- Will you be able to operate your equipment safely in the provided space without risk of injury?
- Create a list of additional special supplies that you will need in this environment, including first aid, personal protective equipment, etc.
- Is there control of noise and telephones so that they do not interfere with the treatment?
- Is there control of children or pets so that they do not interfere with the treatment?
- What will be the source of clean water for use in the treatment? Have disinfecting wipes so that the cleanliness of this source can be assured.
- If sharps will be involved in the treatment, a sharps container will need to be included in the service checklist. Make provisions for discarding gloves and disposable items contaminated with blood or bodily fluids.
- Make provisions for transporting items such as contaminated instruments and linen after the treatment.
- Make a complete list of all items that will be needed to perform the service, including any sub-items that will be required to do this safely.

Common Accidents and Prevention

Accidents are defined as unplanned events that disrupt normal operations and can result in injury or damage. Every accident will be preceded by an unsafe act

STATE REGULATORY ALERT

Prior to performing any treatment or service off-site, check with your state regulatory agency and insurance agent to confirm legality of working outside the employment facility.

or condition or simply by negligence. Most accidents occur from overlooking a potential hazard or from failing to follow protocols that would prevent or control that hazard.

In the clinic setting, common causes of accidents or injuries may be found in one of several categories:

- Chemicals
- Cross-contamination
- Cuts, scratches, and punctures
- Skin disorders
- Electrical safety
- Repetitive motion and ergonomics
- Fire or burns
- Product spills
- Slip, trip, and fall hazards

Chemicals

Chemicals can cause many types of accidents throughout the clinic, whether they are professional esthetic use products or common cleaning agents. Chemicals can trigger allergic reactions, skin irritation by contact, or respiratory irritation from inhaling vapors or dust. Improper chemical use can cause skin to become overly dry, possibly to the point where it chaps, peels, or cracks. Chemical skin reactions or burns are another hazard and may not be recognized immediately. Adhering to manufacturer instructions, carefully following proper mixing guidelines, and using personal protective equipment are critical. You should always have MSDS sheets readily available on all chemicals and adhere to their recommendations for handling, as they are all irritants and carry risks. It is important to consider all substances to be potentially hazardous chemicals, even if they are commonly used and seem safe (Figure 3–4). Some products, when used incorrectly, may result in overexposure and create a skin response as contact dermatitis with an irritant or allergic reaction.

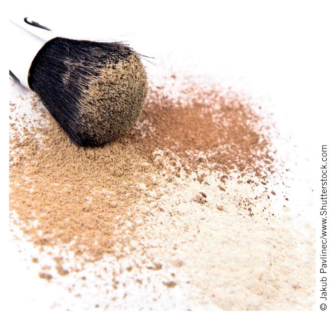

FIGURE 3-4 Avoid inhalations of all chemical agents including cosmetic powders.

© Jakub Pavlinec/www.Shutterstock.com

Cross-Contamination

Cross-contamination is a frequent hazard in the esthetic clinic. Cross-contamination occurs when an object such as the skin is touched, followed by an object or product being touched with the same hand or utensil. A common cause of cross-contamination is in cosmetic application when the chosen applicator tool moves from the original cosmetic product to the skin and is followed by the tool returning to the original container for additional product. Cross-contamination is essentially the transference of contamination from the skin to a product or application tool, or vice versa (Figure 3–5). This type of hazard can come from a client

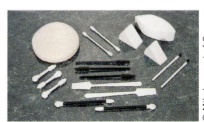

FIGURE 3-5 Disposable cosmetic applicators are one cross contamination prevention method.

© Milady, a part of Cengage Learning. Photography by Larry Hamill.

with a contagious disorder, from unclean implements, from products that are contaminated, from improper dispensing or application of products, or from improper handling of skin where the protective barrier has been compromised. It can also occur from poor sanitation in general. The dispensary, general clinic areas, and every aspect of the treatment area must be properly maintained to prevent cross-contamination. Following stringent infection-control practices will minimize the risk of cross-contamination.

Cuts, Scratches, or Punctures

Cuts, scratches, and punctures are all potential hazards for estheticians and their clients. A break in the skin may come from a simple paper cut, scissors, or tweezers or while using a brow shaper blade. Poorly maintained equipment, too-long fingernails, or an implement could scratch the client's skin. An esthetician may have an infected hangnail, or chapped skin that could unexpectedly crack open. Injuries can also result from a lancet or a poke from scissors, a mascara wand, or a cosmetic brush if a client moves without warning. Other skin abrasions can occur from chemical treatment, waxing, microdermabrasion, or other exfoliation treatments. The result is the same for all of these situations: a breach of the skin's protective barrier.

The use of personal protective equipment like gloves and safety practices such as routine hand washing can minimize risks. Following protocols for the appropriate care and use of implements and the routine maintenance of equipment is also crucial.

Skin Disorders

When dealing with a skin disorder, estheticians must first be able to distinguish distressed skin from a skin disorder or disease. A thorough client consultation and skin analysis is the second phase of offering high-quality treatments (Figure 3–6).

A client who has a contagious condition must be rescheduled to prevent either spreading it on the client's own body or transmitting it to another person. There may be conditions or situations where the best course of action is to refer the client to a medical professional. In this type of situation, communicate this with tact so that the client feels you are concerned about his or her health.

An esthetician is not licensed to diagnose or offer treatments if it appears that a client should seek medical treatment. Often, an esthetician may feel absolutely certain that a client should receive a medical

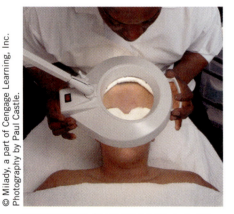

© Milady, a part of Cengage Learning, Inc. Photography by Paul Castle.

FIGURE 3–6 Conducting a thorough skin analysis provides clues to any obscure signs of a skin disorder.

STATE REGULATORY ALERT

In some states, technicians may be allowed to practice dermaplaning, which is exfoliation using a surgical blade for a controlled scraping of dead skin cells. Always check with your local licensing agency about legality prior to offering this type of treatment.

referral, but if you are ever in doubt, consider the following as consideration a client should likely seek medical advisement.

- When any undiagnosed or unidentified rash is present. If any blemish or growth of the skin has been changing, enlarging, or oozing or does not fit into a standard skin blemish category.
- When a client has expectations that are beyond your scope of practice as an esthetician, such as the elimination or removal of age spots.
- Any time you see something unusual on the skin that you are unsure of or do not recognize.

Electrical Safety

Electrical safety attempts to control electrical hazards such as treatments that use electrical currents, electrical shock, and electricity as potential ignition sources. The safety of electrical equipment used in treatments is discussed in more detail in Chapter 4. Reading the safety manual and following the instructions from the manufacturer will explain how to safely use any electrical item. It is sometimes easy to overlook common items as a potential electrical hazard. One example of an electrical hazard is the improper use of a clothes dryer. Laundering linens in a clinic or spa may require use of a washer and dryer. The lint generated from the dryer must be thoroughly removed after every load and the dryer should never be left to run unattended. Vent hoses and areas should be cleaned routinely to prevent lint buildup and a combustible fire hazard.

Another electrical hazard may result from electrical equipment being exposed to water or other chemicals; this includes handling electrical cords or appliances with wet hands. Poorly maintained cords, equipment, and filters all pose potential risks. Reading the safety manuals and following the self-inspection and safety checklists are a major element of controlling electrical hazards.

Product Spills

An accidental product spill can happen anywhere in the clinic (Figure 3–7). A dropped container may be ruptured or broken. All spills, sprays, or splashes pose a risk of eye or skin injury. Products or vapors can also irritate the throat, lungs, or stomach; burn the skin; trigger an allergy; or cause someone to slip or fall. Minimize these risks by keeping containers closed and dispensing products carefully. When using anything that sprays, avoid pointing it at the client's face. Instead, spray horizontally and let it mist down onto the client. This not only is safer but is a softer and more pleasant experience for the client.

When using a toner or other product that contains alcohol or common chemical irritants, avoid spraying it. For toners, select products with a flip top and apply them to a cotton pad or gauze square for application. If you are dealing with a cleaning agent, hold the container at hip height and spray it onto a paper towel

> **CAUTION**
>
> If using an airbrush device to apply facial makeup, make sure that the spray power does not exceed 6 to 8 pounds of pressure per square inch; this will generally be termed the PSI. Eye injuries have been reported at higher pressure levels. For body work, the pressure may be increased and should range from 9 to 15 PSI.

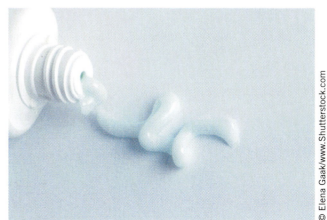

FIGURE 3–7 Safe practices include cleaning up all spills immediately.

© Elena Gaak/www.Shutterstock.com

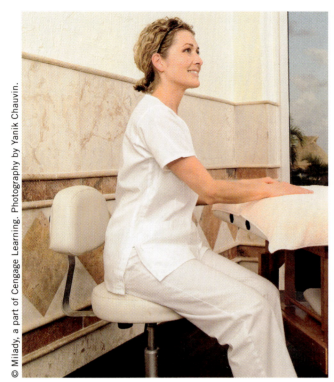

FIGURE 3–8 Use of a wheeled stool will assist ergonomic body adjustment to the height of the work surface.

© Milady, a part of Cengage Learning. Photography by Yanik Chauvin.

or other applicator. This will minimize your inhaling vapors or particulates. These recommendations may apply even to common cleaning agents if you review the directions for use or MSDS sheets.

Slip, Trip, and Fall Hazards

Clinic hazards in this category generally occur from poor housekeeping habits or obstructed walkways. Boxes, cabinets, shelving, and other objects should not be stored where they may create a traffic hazard. We need to be aware of treatment particulates that can cause a floor to become slippery. Powders and granules can turn a floor into an extremely slick surface. Oils, wax, water, and any other product that spills should be cleaned up immediately to protect both the technician and the client. Clients receiving body services should be provided with safe footwear to move from one area to another.

Attractive flooring choices found in today's facilities can also pose risks. Wet tile, marble, and other materials can be particularly slippery both to bare feet and to shoes without slip-resistant soles. All employers of estheticians should include in their safety plans provisions for safe and sanitary footwear choices.

Repetitive Motion and Ergonomics

The use of repeated motions and failure to practice proper ergonomics will create risks for the technician and the staff. Incorrect posture and movements can cause injury resulting in lost work or even loss of a career (Figure 3–8). After a busy day, many technicians have felt the effects of fatigue and muscle or tendon irritation. Left unchecked, over time and repeated use, these can progress and develop into debilitating strains or sprains. Proper ergonomics may not come naturally and must be practiced with a focus on numerous factors.

Here are some questions you may ask yourself when conducting an examination of factors affecting ergonomics:

- Is the working surface too high, too low, or too far away?
- What range of motion and how much force must be used?
- What position or posture is required for the task and can it be made more ergonomic?
- Is repeated motion required?
- Is the motion constant, or are breaks or pauses possible?
- Do you have to use the "flag" position? (This is bending forward at the waist at about a 45° angle, one of the angles most likely to generate back strain.)
- Do you have to reach horizontally with heavy items?
- Do you stand in one position for an extended time?
- Do you sit for a lengthy timeframe?
- Will you be doing anything that involves awkward or uncomfortable positions?

Fire or Burns

Fire safety is an important concern in every clinic, salon, and spa. Electrical issues have already been discussed, but there are other contributing factors, as well. All potential for burns must be evaluated and plans made to control the risk. Burning candles have been eliminated in many facilities due to their high risk. Non-flame candle-type devices or specialty lamps can create ambiance and offer a safer alternative.

Other burn sources could include chemicals and overheated stones, water, or towels. Chemical burns may come from glycolic peels or other acidic products. Always monitor potential sources of chemical burns such as glycolic and lactic acids closely. All sources for potential chemical or physical burns should be identified and protocols established. Showers should be equipped with safety mechanisms to prevent sudden changes in water temperature when additional pull on the water resources is created.

The dispensary should also be evaluated to ensure that products are appropriately stored to prevent combustion. Containers should be kept closed to prevent vapor buildup. Products containing alcohol, acetone, or other flammable liquids should not be stored near any heat source and should be kept away from combustibles such as fabric, wood, paper, or cardboard.

Accident Prevention

Preventing accidents is always important. Having a plan prior to an accident occurring will be helpful by minimizing stress so that proper care can be given. Common terms used for this type of plan include "Accident Prevention Program" or "Safety and Health Plan." This could be a written plan of elements important to accident prevention. Some components that should be included in your plan are listed below.

- Safety orientation
- A description of your total safety and health program
- On-the-job orientation showing employees what they need to know to perform their initial job assignments safely
- How and when to report on-the-job injuries, including instruction about the location of first-aid facilities in your workplace (Figure 3-9)
- How to report unsafe conditions and practices
- The use and care of required personal protective equipment (PPE)
- What to do in an emergency, including how to exit the workplace
- Identification of hazardous gases, chemicals, or materials used on the job and instruction about safe use and the emergency action to take after accidental exposure

STATE REGULATORY ALERT

Know your state guidelines on the usage of chemical peels. A wide variation exists from state to state concerning the types of chemicals permitted, the recommended strengths, and other factors.

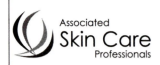

Claim Form
General Liability Loss Notice
Business Personal Property Loss Notice

Insured

Name:_____ ASCP ID No. _____

Address: _____ City:_____ State: _____ Zip:_____

Home: (   ) _____ Work: (   )_____

Name of Person to Contact: _____

Address: _____ City:_____ State: _____ Zip:_____

Home: (   ) _____ Work: (   )_____

Best time to reach: _____ ❑ am ❑ pm   E-mail address: _____

Loss (Business Personal Property Claims only)

Location of Accident (include city, state & zip): _____

_____

Date of Loss: ___/___/___   Time of Loss:_____❑ am ❑ pm   Previously reported to ASCP? ❑ Yes ❑ No

Authority Contacted: _____

Brief Description of Accident (attach detailed report)_____

_____

Injured/Property Damaged   Date of Injury/Damage_____

Name of Injured/Owner of Damaged Property:_____

Address: _____ City:_____ State: _____ Zip:_____

Phone: (   )_____ Age:_____ Gender: ❑ M ❑ F Occupation: _____

E-mail: _____

Employer's Name: _____

Address: _____ City:_____ State: _____ Zip:_____

E-mail: _____

Telephone: (   ) _____ Fatality? ❑ Yes ❑ No

Briefly describe what injured was doing/injury/damage (attach detailed report) _____

_____

Witnesses

Name:_____ E-mail _____

Address: _____ City:_____ State: _____ Zip:_____

Home: (   ) _____ Work: (   )_____

Remarks: _____

_____

Name:_____ E-mail _____

Address: _____ City:_____ State: _____ Zip:_____

Home: (   ) _____ Work: (   )_____

Remarks: _____

_____

FIGURE 3–9 Insurance report form.

Other Insurance Coverage

It is important you include copies of any and all certificates of insurance you may hold for professional liability insurance coverage or business liability coverage, whether through other association affiliations or independent agents.

Company Name:_____

Contact: _____

Address: _____

City: _____ State: _____ Zip: _____

Policy No. _____ Phone: (_____) _____

Comments/Description

_____

_____

_____

_____

_____

_____

_____

_____

_____

_____

_____

_____

_____

Signature of Insured

Signature:_____ Date:_____

Associated Skin Care Professionals

submit to
ASCP Risk Management Coordinator
1271 Sugarbush Drive, Evergreen, Colorado 80439
800-789-0411
fax 800-790-0299
getconnected@ascpskincare.com
www.ascpskincare.com

ASCP 02/08

FIGURE 3–9 Insurance report form. (continued)

- Provision of regular in-service and continuing education
- Annual evaluation of employee safety practices

However, no amount of preparedness can prevent all accidents. In the event of an accident, it may become important for you to show that you have made efforts in prevention. Risk management may offer a broader understanding.

RISK MANAGEMENT

During the course of conducting our business, we will encounter some inherent risks. Risk management is about controlling and minimizing these potential dangers. The first thing we must do is to recognize, acknowledge, and understand these risks. We also need to know what to do to reduce these risks in our day-to-day operations. Reduction of risk can be accomplished by making efforts to minimize, monitor, and control the likelihood of possible accidents occurring.

Risk management is a broad term. It may not be entirely clear in its definition or what it encompasses. The National Coalition of Esthetic Alliances (NCEA) defines risk management for the esthetics industry as the recognition of risk, risk assessment, developing strategies to manage risk, and mitigation of risk using managerial resources.

Strategies an esthetician may use for risk management include prevention or avoidance of risk, reducing the negative effect of the risk, and accepting some or all of the consequences of a specific risk. Some traditional risk management elements focus on risks stemming from physical, natural, or legal concerns. Some examples of this include natural disasters, fires, accidents, injury or death, and lawsuits. Besides careful planning and prevention, another essential component of risk management is making sure you are covered by professional liability insurance.

Liability Coverage

Liability is defined as the legal responsibility for something, especially costs or damages. It is in your best interest to hold personal and/or business liability coverage. Accidents may happen at any time and cannot always be prevented. Maintaining proper liability coverage may prove beneficial when a client has an adverse response or sudden allergic reaction. It is essential that you be protected if faced with a legal dispute. More information specific to your area can be found through your professional organizations, training school, small business associations, and local insurance agency (Figure 3–10).

Carrying appropriate professional liability insurance is crucial for all practicing estheticians. When purchasing or using new equipment or offering a new treatment or additional types of services, you should make sure to review your current policies with your agent. You may need to upgrade or change your current insurance coverage. The type of liability coverage and how much you carry may be determined by your licensing board. It is suggested that you develop a good relationship with your agent and always carry ample coverage.

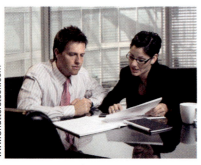

© Zsolt Nyulaszi/
www.Shutterstock.com

FIGURE 3-10 Personally meet with your insurance representative to discuss details of coverage.

Legal Risk Management

In order to function as an esthetician, you must generally be licensed or certified in your state (or country). Achieving this status should be taken seriously and will require that you possess proper knowledge and understand that you are expected to follow only the allowed scope of practice. Your state regulatory board issues guidelines or scope of practice rules that you, as a licensee, are required to abide by. It is your responsibility to seek out the state regulations and keep yourself updated. In some cases, a change in a law may greatly affect your daily practice of esthetics.

Under most legal systems, you have a duty of care toward your clients. This is the legal obligation imposed, stating that when you as a licensed professional provide a service, you are expected to work with a reasonable standard of care. If a client is unaware of an allergy, it could present risk of serious harm or death—as in the case of anaphylactic shock. If the client is aware of his or her allergies but we do not inquire about them, then we are not practicing legal risk management.

Negligence, in most legal systems, is the failure to meet the standard of expected care. In the event of an accident or adverse reaction to a client, legal action may be sought by the client based on your negligence. This is called a lawsuit or being sued. The client—the plaintiff in the suit—may claim that you failed to meet the standard of care and were negligent in your treatment, and that that negligence led to the injury-causing accident. You would then be responsible for hiring your own legal representation and could be held liable. If you are found to be the responsible party for the injury, you may owe for damages as determined by the court, as well as jeopardizing the status of your licensure. Obviously, avoidance of legal risk can be accomplished by always working with caution and preparedness.

FYI

Your most important obligation in managing legal risk is to use your best efforts to avoid foreseeable accidents or adverse reactions while operating within your scope of practice.

Steps of Risk Management in the Event of an Accident

There are common incidents that occur in an esthetic environment. A client reading a magazine in your waiting room could get a paper cut. In this situation, the simple use of first aid and a bandage will suffice. During the course of professionally administered treatments, however, accidents can and will happen. Sometimes an accident may be more severe or even require medical assistance. In this situation, being mentally prepared will help you think more clearly. How you manage the accident and attendant circumstances can make all the difference in the case of a lawsuit and help determine whether you are found to be legally at fault. A few things to consider in the event that this type of unfortunate situation occurs include:

1. The first priority is handling the incident. Depending on the procedure and what you are doing at the time of the accident, your immediate attention and action to prevent further injury may be required. NCEA recommends that all professionals have Emergency First Aid Provider or First Aid/CPR and AED certifications and be able to act quickly to avert further harm to the client. If you are administering CPR, call for assistance and have them contact emergency medical care immediately.

2. Show compassion and do everything possible for the well-being of the client. If possible, inform the client's spouse or emergency contact person. This information should be readily available on the Client Consultation Form.

3. Cooperate with authorities and medical personnel and provide them with all facts of the accident.

4. Do not assign, admit to, or speculate on causes or blame. This detracts from managing the accident and assisting the client. Second, do not provide incomplete and/or inaccurate information. Statements made concerning the cause of an accident may be misunderstood or used against you if legal action is pursued.

5. Make sure that all of the client's belongings are gathered and turned over to the authorities or to the client's emergency contact person.

6. Contact your local insurance agent or the company and complete an Incident Report form. Your facility may also have a policy in place that requires additional incident or first aid reports; if the accident involved a coworker, there may be worker compensation claims reports to file, as well. If you are unable to acquire these forms quickly, it will be helpful to document the incident in writing as soon as possible. Crucial information to include would be the date, time, and location of the incident, who was involved, what treatments were in progress, and any possible contributing factors.

Safety in the clinic requires evaluation, planning and following protocols and techniques for managing potential risks and hazards. Always be aware of what federal and state standards you must comply with, as well as contributing factors for common accidents, prevention, and risk management. Being a professional means making an effort to notice details and investing your time in developing the necessary plans for protecting your clients and yourself.

Equipment Safety

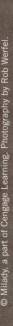

INTRODUCTION

Equipment safety requires attentive and consistent care, including inspection, maintenance, and proper handling. Equipment safety begins with selecting safe equipment then following manufacturer instructions for both safe operation and maintenance. There may be special cleaning involved, wiring to check, and tips, blades, or other components that must be inspected routinely. Various components such as tubes or filters may need to be replaced periodically; replacement parts must be ordered in a timely fashion. The process is completed by ensuring that the use of the equipment is appropriate for the client and that it is operated in a manner that will cause no harm to the client or technician.

SELECT SAFE EQUIPMENT

Commonly, equipment may be purchased by estheticians based on a sales demonstration. This type of equipment purchase is due to commercial or market appeal and the appearance of the sales demonstration. Solid analysis and comparison of equipment is a more business-like approach that will yield better results.

When shopping for equipment, ensuring that the manufacturer has followed specific guidelines will provide confidence in the equipment's safe operation. The National Coalition of Estheticians, Manufacturers/Distributors and Associations (NCEA) has created an equipment evaluation form that is available on their Web site, www.ncea.tv/ns/standards.html, for free download (Figure 4–1). This useful form provides questions to ask to make sure the supplier has followed national safety standards. A condensed version of considerations prior to purchasing equipment is listed here.

- Is the company stable?
- Will the company or representatives be available for support?
- Does the manufacturer provide training?
- What forms and documentation are provided with the equipment?
- If repairs are needed, is this easily accomplished?
- Is equipment available while repairs are being completed?
- Has the wiring been inspected?
- What are the safety precautions when operating the equipment?
- What is cost of treatment performed with the equipment?
- What components need to be replaced and at what cost and frequency?
- What are the indications and contraindications associated with this equipment?
- Is the technology involved within my scope of practice (can it be legally used in my state under my license)?

Researching the warranty of the product can often provide clues as to the quality of production and support you can anticipate from the company. Sometimes a less expensive unit may result in a much higher cost over time much if the equipment requires frequent maintenance or replacements of parts. A lengthy lifespan or warranty for one piece of equipment will not transfer to a different piece or type of equipment. Networking with other estheticians is a good way to find brands that operate safely and have a good lifespan.

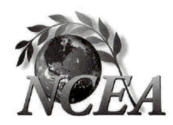

National Coalition of Esthetic & Related Associations
EQUIPMENT EVALUATION FORM

In keeping with the mission of the NCEA to represent and protect the esthetic and related professions and to convey proper standards of practice, the NCEA has developed a list of questions to consider when evaluating equipment. *By providing this information, the NCEA does not endorse or warrant any equipment, or manufacturer, either express or implied.*

EQUIPMENT IDENTIFICATION AND INFORMATION

Name of equipment:

Type of equipment:

Model number:

Price:

What is the manufacturers 'Intended Use Statement'?

Company profile information:

Sales Contact Information:

Name:

Address:

City: State: Zip:

Tel:

Fax:

Email:

Website:

Length of time in business:

Distributor Contact Information:

Name:

Address:

City: State: Zip:

Tel:

Fax:

Email:

Website:

Length of time in business:

Notes:

REGISTRATIONS / CERTIFICATIONS

Is the manufacturer registered with the FDA?

If yes, what is the registration number?

Is the equipment registered with the FDA?

If yes, what is the registration number and class?

Is the device registered with the state, if required?

SAFETY CONSIDERATIONS AND EQUIPMENT SPECIFICATIONS

What safety certifications does this equipment have (i.e. UL, CSA, CE)?

What kind of power source does the equipment require?

Does the manufacturer carry product liability insurance on this equipment?

Is a certificate of insurance available?

Does the equipment have any cross-contamination safeguards, if applicable?

What are the contraindications for use of this equipment?

If purchasing a used device,
  a) What was the date of the last preventative maintenance?
  b) Is the preventative maintenance report available?

WARRANTY AND SERVICE POLICIES

What are the terms of the warranty?

Is there an extended warranty available?

Is there an additional cost?

Do you have an equipment loaner program?

Are references available?

TRAINING AND EDUCATION

What type of training is included with purchase?

Where?   Total hours?

Who are the educators?

Is there an additional cost?

Skin care professionals are required to check in their state as to whether training on the use of equipment is required prior to purchasing, and/or if they can use device under their scope of practice.

To join the NCEA and for Additional Position Papers
go online to www.ncea.tv

FIGURE 4–1 NCEA Equipment Evaluation Form.

Some equipment may have plastic outer casings and LED (light-emitting diode) readout displays; not all of these hold up to exposure to high-level disinfecting agents. Find out from the manufacturer what can be used on these areas to ensure they are properly disinfected. Maintaining the equipment manual from the manufacturer is important to the safe operation of equipment. Be sure to ask the vendor what directions and instructions are included with the device.

FOLLOW MANUFACTURER DIRECTIONS GUIDELINES

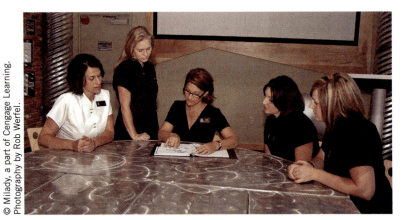

FIGURE 4–2 All employees should read equipment manuals.

© Milady, a part of Cengage Learning. Photography by Rob Werfel.

Take the time to carefully read the manual that comes with a piece of equipment and learn about its safe operation and maintenance (Figure 4–2). Every device is slightly different, and spending a few minutes with the manual can prevent accidents, make using equipment more efficient, and increase the equipment's lifespan. With the new technologies that are coming to market every year, there can be quite a variation in use from one brand to another. For example, one facial toning device may have you hold each position for 2 seconds, while another requires you to hold it longer.

It is critical to always follow manufacturer's guidelines when selecting modalities and products for treatments. This is crucial to protecting the client, which is the ultimate responsibility of the operator as mandated by state and national regulations. Some state regulations may be very general; others are more specific for different types of equipment.

The problems that have been reported to insurance agencies, state regulatory boards, or legal councils are generally cases where manufacturer guidelines were not adequately understood or followed. Other problems include incomplete client history forms or inadequate training of the technician in the treatment to be performed. These are all considered to be negligence on the part of the technician. Negligence can have a number of negative outcomes: injury to a client, loss of career, and/or severe financial loss.

Never overlook small details in your desire to get quick results or accommodate a busy schedule. For example, esthetic equipment might say not to perform a chemical peel following a microdermabrasion treatment; if a technician chooses to perform a peel despite manufacturer warnings, the technician alone is responsible for any negative results. A reaction could lead to a lawsuit even though the client may have signed a consent form. A technician who wishes to combine protocols must verify with both the product manufacturer and the equipment manufacturer that it is safe to do so. This should be in writing so that the technician has the documentation in case of future issues.

It is common practice for a manufacturer to recommend that specific products be used with an equipment modality. These are most often the products that they have used to test the equipment. If questioned about use with other products, the manufacturer most often will reply that the "equipment was not tested with those products." This means that they cannot predict a result and are uncertain how the skin may respond. Sometimes this may be a sales or marketing tool; sometimes it is based on clinical research. It takes careful questions to determine the facts and choose the best course of action.

It is necessary for estheticians to protect themselves. If you do not follow manufacturer guidelines and there is a problem, you may be faced with liability, litigation, and loss of insurance support. Being knowledgeable about the proper use of professional equipment allows for equipment dependability and a more predictable result.

EQUIPMENT MAINTENANCE AND SAFE USE

Maintenance is a major component of equipment safety and is just as important as practicing safe equipment use. Every piece of equipment needs to be checked and routine maintenance performed. There is nothing more frustrating that attempting to use a device in a treatment and discovering a problem. A chart for checking and maintaining equipment can be helpful so that nothing is forgotten. Some equipment will need to go on a daily list, and others only weekly or monthly based on use. Some types of equipment will need specific care.

Treatment Lounge

There are many variations in size and type of treatment lounges used in the salon or spa. Some are massage tables, others are fixed-height treatment beds, and others may incorporate manual or power hydraulics to facilitate use (Figure 4–3). The bed should be selected with consideration for several factors:

- **Size:** Will it fit in the space available with room to get around it?
- **Weight capacity:** Will it accommodate clients comfortably and safely?
- **Treatments to be offered:** Will it accommodate facials, waxing, and body treatments?
- **Materials:** Is the cover sturdy medical-grade vinyl for longevity?
- **Safety:** What safety factors are integrated into it?
- **Height:** Will it allow you to perform all services with ergonomic safety?

Treatment bed maintenance includes surface disinfection after every client and doing a routine safety inspection. The insurance industry reports that accidents have occurred when an adjusting bar gave way and the back of the bed dropped unexpectedly. All components of the bed should be inspected daily to ensure safe client use. Massage tables often have knobs that lock the legs into height position. These knobs can work loose over time or even fall off, leaving the leg at risk for detaching from the bed. Completing a daily check that all hardware is secure and adjustable components are working properly is a brief and simple process. Considerations to include on an equipment checklist for a treatment lounge:

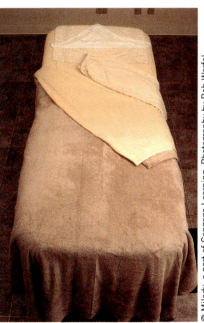

FIGURE 4–3 Prepared treatment bed.

© Milady, a part of Cengage Learning. Photography by Rob Werfel.

- Is the cover material intact and in good repair?
- Are all adjusting knobs and screws secure?
- Are all adjustable portions working properly?
- If hydraulic, is the canister sound and not leaking?
- **Clean:** Is the entire bed, including the base, clean and in good repair?

Magnifying Lamp

The magnifying lamp, also commonly referred to as a mag lamp or loupe, is an essential tool for every esthetician (Figure 4–4). This piece of equipment employs a cool fluorescent bulb that resides inside a protective plastic cover on the underside of the lamp. Because the light is quite bright, client eye protection is recommended during use.

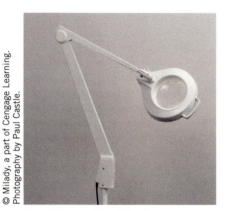

The glass portion of the lamp is a magnifier, the most popular being a 5-diopter lens that provides 50 times magnification power. The lens should be clear and free of any distortion. This is something that should be thoroughly inspected at the time of purchase.

Some lamps may be attached to a rolling stand, while others are attached to a multifunction device or are clamp-on units. The choice for which unit will depend on the individual room setup. Inspect the lamp for adjustable components such as knobs, dials, or hinges. Adjustable components may need to be loosened any time an adjustment is to be made to lamp placement. If this is not done correctly, the lamp head must be forced into position, causing undue wear and tear on the adjusters. The result is a lamp that will fall out of position unexpectedly or that will no longer hold a fixed position. This creates a safety hazard for both client and technician.

The lamp and arm should be disinfected by wiping them down with high-level disinfectant. If the lamp is on a rolling stand, this also requires routine cleaning. Be sure to clean and disinfect both the top and the bottom side of the lens. Once the lamp has been disinfected, the lens can be wiped down with a glass cleaner to leave it streak-free and minimize the risk of eyestrain during use.

Numerous tiny screws hold the light cover in place. These should be checked to make sure they have not loosened. Periodically, the lamp may need to be replaced. The lamps can be purchased at a specialty lighting store.

FIGURE 4-4 Magnifying lamp.

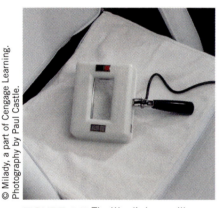

FIGURE 4-5 The Wood's lamp will expose skin problems that may not be visible to the naked eye.

Wood's Lamp

The Wood's lamp is a specialty magnifier that uses filtered black light to illuminate fungi, bacterial disorders, pigmentation, and so on (Figure 4–5). Safety protocols for a Wood's lamp include protecting the client's eyes during use. The lamp should be disinfected after use, following manufacturer directions, and the lens treated like any fine glass magnifier. Never use paper towels to clean the lens, as this may produce small scratches or etching.

Hot Towel Cabinet

Hot towel cabinets come in a variety of sizes and configurations (Figure 4–6). They must be kept clean and free of mold or mildew. After each use, wipe

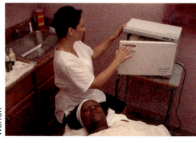

FIGURE 4-6 A hot towel cabinet is used in many forms of esthetic treatment.

the interior of the cabinet with a surface disinfectant and do a thorough cleaning inside and out at the end of the day. Always leave the door open at night to allow the interior and the seals to dry completely. Check the water collection tray underneath the cabinet and empty and clean it on a daily basis. Thermostats may malfunction over time and should be monitored; regularly check electrical cords for fraying.

Steamer

Steamers are available in many styles and capabilities. Steamers may come with ozone features, but this is not found on all models. Certain types of steamers have provisions for infusions of herbs or essential oils. To avoid accident or injury, only add essential oils or herbs for units designed to hold them. Never place this type of additive directly into the water, as this can result in spitting or jar breakage. Some steamers may have a replaceable wick-type filter at the opening of the nozzle. If you wish to use essential oils, place one or two drops on the wick prior to turning the steamer on. The steamer should be placed behind the client or to the side; the steamer arm should be no closer than 16 inches to the client's face (Figure 4–7).

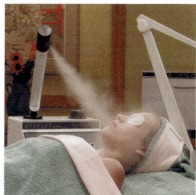

FIGURE 4–7 Place the steamer nozzle a approximately 16 inches from the face.

When placing the water jar on the steamer unit, make sure it is well seated in the ring and that the support knob that keeps the jar in position is properly tightened; never over-tighten. Glass expands and contracts with temperature changes; if the knob is too tight, it can cause the glass to crack or break when heated.

When turning on the steamer, never turn on the ozone unit until the steam is being released through the arm nozzle. Never leave any steamer unattended while heating. It is easy to be away longer than anticipated and the steamer could run low on water, causing glass breakage. Always follow the fill lines on the jar and keep in mind that not all steamers have automatic shutoff systems.

After each use, disinfect the exterior of the steamer. The jar should be emptied every night, thoroughly rinsed, and allowed to dry. The rubber seal along the rim of the jar must also be kept clean. Use only distilled water to prevent the coils from becoming corroded. Buildup can also occur if water is left standing in the jar overnight or for extended periods of time.

The steamer should be cleaned frequently. A steamer that is emitting steam, spits, or drips may need to be cleaned. Spitting can cause injury to clients should it land on their skin.

Steamer Cleaning

Cleaning is best done in a well-ventilated area due to the odor of the vinegar.

1. Place 2 tablespoons of white vinegar in the steamer jar. Fill jar to the maximum level with distilled water.
2. Turn on steamer and let it heat until steam is produced. Do not turn on an ozone feature.
3. Allow steamer to steam for 20 minutes or until the water level drops to the low-level indicator.
4. Turn off the steamer and allow it to stand for 15 minutes or until the unit has cooled. Do not attempt to handle a hot container.

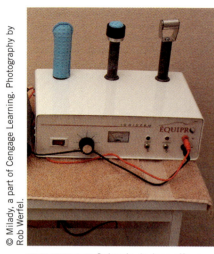

FIGURE 4–8 Galvanic devices offer a variety of electrode types.

5. Once the unit has cooled, empty the water jar completely and rinse well. Replace in the steamer unit, refill with clean distilled water, and heat to steaming.

6. Allow the steamer to operate for about 10 minutes. If an odor remains, repeat steps 4 and 5.

Never leave cleaning solution in the steamer overnight, as it can corrode the coils and damage the unit. Most steamers have a reset button on the back of the device. If you have trouble with normal operation, check the reset button.

Galvanic Device

The galvanic device is commonly offered in treatments of deincrustation and iontophoresis (Figure 4–8). This type of device is relatively trouble-free and easy to maintain. General, regular cleaning begins with powering the device off and disconnecting the electrode from the power source. Properly dispose of any soiled cotton or sponge components. Separate all removable parts and treat individually. Never soak the electrode unless the manufacturer specifically advises to do so; liquid may penetrate the electrode and damage electrical components. Never process the electrode in an autoclave, as the heat will destroy the internal wiring. Plastic or rubber gaskets may be detached and soaked in a germicidal solution for 10 minutes. The metal tips of rollers can be removed and immersed in disinfectant for the required time. The electrode should be wiped down with a hospital-strength disinfectant after each use. Do not neglect to review and follow specific guidelines from the manufacturer for cleaning and disinfecting.

On a daily basis, the casing of the galvanic device should be cleaned according to the manufacturer's guidelines. Knobs and switches that are used for machine adjustment should be wiped down with a disinfectant between uses.

For galvanic safety, always turn the current to the lowest level when the machine is being turned off and maintain this level when not in use. Confirm that the client has removed jewelry from the hand preferred for holding the electrode; this is generally the dominant hand. This minimizes current crossing the heart area. Always place the electrode that is to be used on the client directly against the client's skin before turning on the device. Some galvanic devices may have both a power setting switch and a current adjustment; others may have a single knob. Power on the current and then slowly adjust the current level to one that is comfortable for the client. Maintain constant contact during the procedure and continually move the electrode. You may use your free hand to add more moisture to the skin as necessary to facilitate the proper slide. When the treatment is complete, turn the current down, turn the power off, and then remove the electrode from the skin.

Galvanic current should not be used on couperose skin, pustular acne, or inflamed areas; on clients who are pregnant or epileptic; or on clients who have pacemakers, heart problems, high blood pressure, or braces. Be sure to know all of the contraindications for using a machine before implementing it in treatments. The client should avoid contact with metal during electrical machine treatments. A burn may occur if contact is made.

Consider taking a hands-on class in galvanic current if it was not covered in your training. The hands-on experience will enhance confidence that the treatment is being performed safely and achieving the desired results.

High-Frequency

High-frequency machines are an excellent method of cleansing, stimulating circulation, and relaxing the skin. This type of machine by glass electrodes attached to a power source to create a high-frequency or sinusoidal current. During the manufacturing process, the glass electrodes are filled with neon or argon gas. The type of gas controls the colored glow that is emitted during the treatment. Electrodes come in a variety of shapes, depending on what type of treatment each is to be used for (Figure 4–9). Safety measures include having the client remove jewelry prior to the treatment. The technique employed will depend on whether the treatment is to be performed using direct or indirect techniques. In either case, the applicator should be placed on the skin prior to turning on the current. The current should be adjusted to a comfortable level for the client. When the treatment is completed, leave the applicator in contact with the skin until the current is turned down and powered off.

The thin glass electrodes are fragile and should be stored in a protective wrapping to prevent breakage. After use, they should be wiped down with soap and water. Because of the gas inside, do not use alcohol on high-frequency electrodes. Never immerse the electrode directly into water. The glass tip (not the metal end) may be decontaminated by immersing in a disinfectant following manufacturer directions. Electrodes should never be placed in an autoclave or ultraviolet machine. Properly store the clean electrodes in a clean and covered container.

If, over a period of time, the unit seems to be operating more weakly or losing power, check the manual from the manufacturer to see if the high-frequency coil may need replacement.

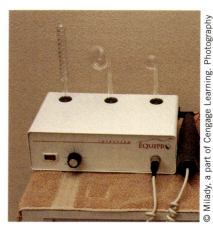

FIGURE 4–9 High frequency devices offer various electrodes, each are used for unique features and benefits.

Spray and Vacuum Devices

The two components of spray and vacuum devices are often sold as a single unit with dual capabilities (Figure 4–10). They have been used in the esthetic industry for many years. The spray component is useful in removing products and eliminating residues, while the vacuum component will increase blood circulation and loosen comedones for removal.

Sprayers

The sprayer is attached to the base unit by means of a flexible hose. The unattached end has a small plastic or glass bottle with a spray nozzle. To use this, the technician turns on the power and places one finger over the vacuum hole to complete the suction circuit; spray will emit from the bottle. Use of a sprayer may cause a client to hold his or her breath due to the continuous flow on the face; safe practices will limit spray time or interrupt the spray so that the client may relax and take a few breaths. Instruct clients to keep their eyes and mouth closed during the process; you may also direct clients to raise a hand to indicate if they need a break.

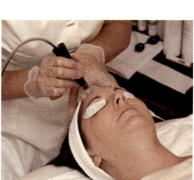
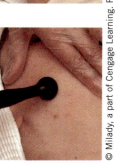

FIGURE 4–10 The spray/vacuum apparatus.

As a safety measure, disconnect the sprayer from the hose when not in use. Store it in such a way that it will not leak and create spills. Sprayers should be wiped down with a disinfecting solution after every use. Follow the manufacturer's cleaning directions and replace the liquid frequently. Flush the sprayer regularly with distilled water to ensure that there is no buildup, and clean at least monthly to prevent a mineral buildup in the nozzle.

Lucas Sprayer

This is a specialized form of sprayer that can be used with warm or cool water. It may also incorporate plant extracts, herbal teas, fresheners, or astringents. It is important to follow the guidelines in the equipment manual for cleaning and disinfecting between product types to assure continued operation (Figure 4–11). It is critical to make sure that the water level is always visible on the water gauge to prevent damage to the device.

Vacuum Device

A vacuum device is another form of the sprayer and vacuum unit. The vacuum is attached to the base unit with slender tubing. At the end that is not attached to the unit, various glass or metal suction cups may be connected. This device is not designed to remove quantities of product from the skin; attempts to use it for that purpose will likely clog the hose.

Locate the vacuum filter, which is normally located at the end of the hose where it attaches to an opening on the machine. Find out from the supplier about replacement filters, as they may have to be changed frequently. Without a filter, all waste components will gather on the inside of the machine, providing a breeding area for bacteria. Clean or replace the filter according to the equipment manual.

All glass and metal cups or tips should be washed in soap and water, then immersed in hospital-grade disinfectant for the recommended time. Follow the manufacturer's guidelines for cleaning hand pieces and hoses. Protocol should be used to thoroughly clean any potential residue of microorganisms or skin debris from the components between uses. The machine exterior should be kept clean and all dials or switches should be disinfected during the normal cleanup routine after each use.

Lymphatic Drainage Vacuum

The lymphatic drainage vacuum is a specialized form of vacuum device that uses suction massage for lymphatic drainage (Figure 4–12). This type of equipment consists of a base unit with tubes attached to the device housing and glass suction cups attached to the free end by use of a rubber gripper. The suction is not to be used for product removal. This may be used in facial or body treatments with the cups available in different sizes. Following each treatment, the glass cups should be washed in soap and water and immersed in hospital-grade disinfectant. Follow the instructions of the manufacturer on disinfection methods for all rubber or plastic components and tubes. Replace filters in accordance with manufacturer guidelines.

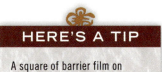

HERE'S A TIP

A square of barrier film on dials or switches provides excellent protection from cross-contamination and speeds up the cleanup process.

© Milady, a part of Cengage Learning. Photography by Rob Werfel.

FIGURE 4–11 Proper use of a Lucas sprayer.

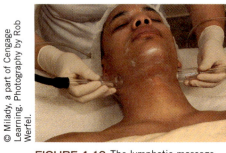

© Milady, a part of Cengage Learning. Photography by Rob Werfel.

FIGURE 4–12 The lymphatic massage device allows you to work on both sides of the face simultaneously.

When using this type of equipment, allow your client to relax prior to treatment and make sure your client is comfortable and kept warm. Cover any exposed body areas that are not being treated. You may apply a fine oil to allow for easy glide and avoid drag on the skin. Prior to applying the vacuum treatment to the client, you may check the degree of pressure on yourself. Do not exceed a 10 percent lift into the cup. If the pressure is excessive, you should adjust as necessary by turning down the control dial, choosing a smaller applicator with a smaller opening, or applying the strokes more quickly by reducing the suction buildup. Avoid using this vacuum with excess lift, as this is uncomfortable for the client and may cause bruising.

Rotary Brushes

An electronic rotary brush may be used for deep cleansing or light exfoliation (Figure 4–13). Safe usage of a brush device depends on proper brush selection and following the manufacturer's recommendations. Brushes should be made from natural bristles and not be used on a dry surface of skin. You should prepare the skin by pre-moistening, and the brush should also be moistened prior to usage. Select the firmness of the brush based on client skin type, choosing the softer brushes for more delicate skin and the firmer ones for thicker or oilier skin. Ensure that the brush is properly attached to the base so that it does not come loose during the treatment.

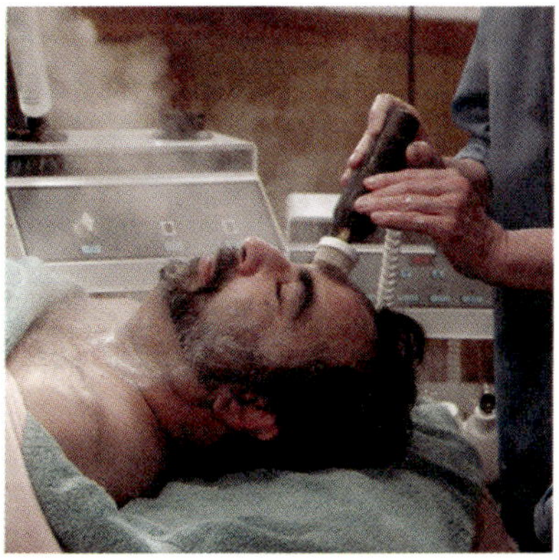

FIGURE 4-13 A rotary brush offers light exfoliation.

To properly care for the brushes, disconnect them from the base and then wash thoroughly with soap and water and rinse well. Immerse the brushes in hospital-strength disinfectant following the manufacturer's guidelines. Rinse thoroughly, air dry, and store properly to avoid contamination.

Handle the brushes carefully so that bristles remain unbent and the shape is not lost during the cleaning and drying process. If the bristles become misshapen, they will not rotate properly and will need immediate replacement. Leaving brushes in an ultraviolet sanitizer can cause the natural fibers to split or break down, resulting in rough, broken ends. As soon as all moisture is gone and the brush is dry, remove the rotary brush and store in a clean and closed container.

Microdermabrasion

Each microdermabrasion unit is configured slightly differently (Figure 4–14). Manufacturer guidelines for maintenance and safe operation should always be diligently read and followed. However, there are some general recommendations when working with this type of unit. All microdermabrasion devices should have the exterior casing wiped down between each treatment. Switches, dials, or other areas that may have been touched with dirty gloves should be properly cleaned with a hospital-strength disinfectant if they were not protected with a square of barrier film. If barrier film is used, it should be properly replaced.

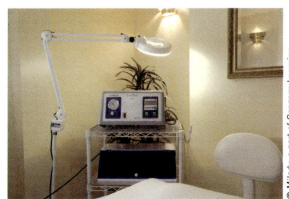

FIGURE 4-14 Crystal microdermabrasion device.

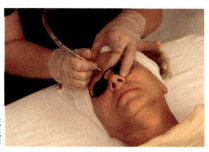

© Milady, a part of Cengage Learning. Photography by Rob Werfel.

FIGURE 4–15 Microdermabrasion treatment with a diamond tip.

The type of tip or tube will vary with each individual device; all of the components must be decontaminated or replaced between uses. Some tips are disposable and should be replaced after each use. Some units allow purchasing of tips for reuse on a single client. The single-client reusable type of tip must be decontaminated after every use following manufacturer guidelines and properly stored and labeled with the name of the client.

All tips should be thoroughly cleaned by removing all product traces and oils prior to immersion in a hospital-strength disinfectant. Metal tips such as the ones found on diamond microdermabrasion units may be processed through an autoclave after they have been properly cleaned (Figure 4–15). Glass tubes should be cleaned and disinfected following guidelines of the manufacturer. Tips or tubes will wear over time and should be routinely inspected to determine if replacement is necessary. Tubes should be cleaned and replaced following manufacturer's recommendations. Microdermabrasion devices may have one or more HEPA filters, and these should be inspected and replaced following manufacturer guidelines.

Devices that use any form of crystal must follow manufacturer and state regulatory guidelines for the handling and disposal of new and used crystals. If manual filling or emptying of a crystal storage area is required, proper personal protective equipment such as a face mask and goggles should be utilized to protect the technician from inhaling the crystal material or getting any into the eyes. Some states require that used crystals be treated as a biohazard material and that appropriate disposal protocols be followed. Local regulatory agencies will be able to offer assistance when any doubts exist concerning proper disposal methods.

To ensure reliable operation of microdermabrasion units, avoid using a steamer in the room where microdermabrasion treatments are offered. The humidity produced by a steamer unit may cause crystal material to cluster together or clump; this may cause a clog in the unit and prevent the machine from operating properly. Using a tip or tube that has any moisture present can also cause clogging within the unit. The skin of the client must be thoroughly dry before starting the procedure, or this too may allow moisture to enter the unit.

Some devices offer the crystals prepackaged in a cartridge that is then installed when the previous one has reached the "too low to use" level. This change should be made prior to beginning a treatment to avoid interruption or any variation in the flow of the crystals. With some units, this cartridge change may require a little time to get the new vial of crystals flowing. Keep the manual handy so that you can troubleshoot in the case of any problems.

To operate a microdermabrasion safely there are several factors to consider:

- Is the treatment appropriate for the client?
- Is the technician wearing personal protective equipment?
- Is the device working properly—appropriate crystal flow?
- Are the client's eyes, nostrils, and ears protected from crystal particulates?
- Are the pressure dial settings correct for the client and the area of the face or body to be worked on?
- Is the pressure being put on the tube/tip correct for the client? (More pressure is more aggressive on diamond-tip devices.) Ask the client to ensure that they are comfortable with the pressure.

- Is the speed of the passes appropriate for the client? Slower is more aggressive on crystal devices, as more crystals hit the same spot of skin. Ask the client to make sure that they are comfortable with the sensation.
- Is the number of passes made over the face appropriate for the client?
- Monitor the skin for signs of redness or irritation to avoid overworking an area.

Ultrasonic

Ultrasonic devices are high-tech units that use high-frequency sonic or sound waves and water to cleanse, exfoliate, and stimulate the skin. When used in a penetration mode, it assists products to penetrate more deeply than can be achieved with manual application.

Estheticians must make sure the device they are using is designed for treatments of the skin and not designed for use in physical therapy treatments. The chief differentiating characteristic between these types of units is the megahertz frequencies. Esthetic devices should offer a 3-megahertz frequency for effective skin use. Slower megahertz frequency units will penetrate too deeply to be useful. Devices with 1-megahertz frequency penetrate 3 to 5 centimeters into the body and can generate heat, discomfort, or even pain. These are commonly used by medical practitioners to treat internal injuries. Always check a new or different device prior to use for the megahertz frequency it generates.

Ultrasonic devices use direct-current electrical units; this requires that some sort of ground be used. General safety will require clients to remove jewelry prior to treatment. If the ground is a separate unit, place it on the client's right wrist or under the right shoulder. Some manufacturers may state that the device can be operated without a ground, but this method will be less effective. Portable devices on the market have small metal bars on each side of the device, which the technician presses as he or she works. In this case, the hand of the technician will act as the ground.

Because they use sound, ultrasonic units emit a soft, high-pitched tone during the exfoliation mode. Some clients may be sensitive to this noise, so you may offer the client cotton or disposable ear plugs to place in the ear. Each modality on the unit generates a different sound. Be sure to advise the client of this prior to the treatment. For clients who have metal dental fillings or implants, the unit can trigger a metallic taste in the mouth or even slight discomfort. Always avoid the eye area, using the orbital bone as a guide and never bringing contact inside of this region. Monitor your client's comfort level at all times and communicate in advance the importance of reporting any discomfort (Figure 4–16).

During exfoliation, the skin should be moist or wet for cavitation to occur. Steaming the skin while doing this step can be helpful. You can use a cotton or gauze pad dipped in distilled water or a wetting solution recommended by the manufacturer to rewet the skin if needed. During the penetration or other available mode, keep the skin moist with serums or products as recommended by the manufacturer. Never work on dry skin, which may cause roughness or drag, resulting in injury.

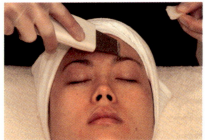

© Milady, a part of Cengage Learning. Photography by Rob Werfel.

FIGURE 4–16 An ultrasonic facial should never be uncomfortable, adjust the settings or discontinue the treatment if necessary.

If working with any form of blade, the edge of the blade should always lightly glide across the skin. Variations in pressure throughout a treatment will interfere with the action of the sound waves. The light touch and nonabrasive nature of the treatment make it useful for more sensitive skin conditions.

Between clients, the exterior case of the device should be wiped down with a manufacturer's recommended solution. Some suggest 70 percent isopropyl alcohol; others suggest use of a high-level disinfectant wipe. Do not use anything abrasive, and keep all liquids away from the joint of the blade and its housing. The blade of the device is made of very thin metal and should be handled like a delicate instrument. Follow manufacturer directions for cleaning and disinfecting between clients and use care in handling to avoid bending, nicking, or pitting the blade.

A damaged blade will not operate correctly. It is easy to determine if a blade is not properly operational. When performing in the exfoliation mode, a fine spray of water should arc away from the blade as it moves across the skin. If this spray is not occurring, the unit is not working properly. The hand piece will then need replacement, while some handheld portable units may need a complete unit replacement.

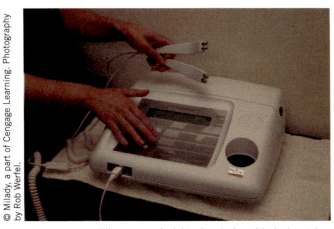

FIGURE 4–17 Microcurrent facial toning device with dual metal probe.

Facial Toning Devices

Toning devices employ two hand pieces that are manipulated on the face to achieve a lifting effect (Figure 4–17). This is accomplished by using a combination of galvanic and faradic current. Use of the proper level of current is critical to receive an optimal result. Estheticians must work with microampere levels of current of .001 or less to be within their scope of practice. True faradic current causes visible muscle contraction and is classified as a medical treatment device.

Microcurrent treatments use gentle electrical stimulation to trigger the body's natural skin enhancement chemicals at a cellular level. This type of treatment is delivered through small hand pieces that may be tipped with a single or double probe. Each probe will end in a small metal sleeve; depending on the manufacturer, either a portion of a cotton swab is inserted into the sleeve or a detachable metal probe is inserted. Always prepare for the treatment by using clean materials and tools. Following each treatment, dispose of cotton properly; if the metal ball probes are used, these should be detached, cleaned, and sterilized. Hand pieces should be wiped down with a disinfectant safe for use on electrical equipment. This type of tool should never be immersed in any liquid so as not to allow liquids to penetrate the hand piece itself. Remember to properly clean the cords and the housing of the device by following manufacturer guidelines.

Each individual client has a different sensitivity to electrical current and each technician may use a slightly different technique or pressure. Always remember to be sure that the client is comfortable with the service being performed and that nothing is causing apprehension or discomfort. Maintain moisture on the skin at all times when performing this technique. Some methods of maintaining the moisture are with the application of steam or the manufacturer-recommended conductive gel or lotion. It may also be necessary to moisten the metal conducting probes or cotton swabs with the manufacturer's product if additional moisture is needed. In addition to toning, some of these devices now also offer the performance of microampere penetration of products or stimulation for cellular homeostasis. Follow manufacturer guidelines for products to be used and technique to be followed, as each brand and type of equipment has unique and slightly different recommendations.

Electrodessication Device

An electrodessication device uses low-level radio-frequency current for the removal of minor skin irregularities. Some units will also offer the ability to incorporate high-frequency; this can arc onto the skin to attract moisture from a lesion. Regulation on these units varies greatly from state to state, but in the majority of states technicians are not allowed to cut, vaporize, or remove skin tissue. These devices are often used to remove skin tags, milia, cholesterol deposits, cherry angiomas, and sebaceous cysts or hyperplasia. It is only logical that such an extreme treatment device may only be used under medical supervision in most states. This type of treatment runs a risk of infection, scarring, hyperpigmentation and hypopigmentation. Proper sterilization must always be performed on this type of equipment prior to use.

LED Lights

LED stands for "light-emitting diode." This type of equipment intends to improve the function and appearance of the skin. These light devices must be disinfected properly to avoid causing any damage to the lights. Prevention of cross-contamination is simplified when the equipment does not make contact with the skin. This is not an issue with some of these devices, as they are on a stand that is lowered to be in close proximity to the client. Some units are handheld; with this type of unit, the distance from the skin means increased amounts of lost energy and possibly unsatisfactory results.

Consult your manufacturer for guidelines as to suggested distance from the skin and acceptable barrier methods to prevent cross-contamination. For some devices, it may be as simple as covering the light probe with a clear plastic barrier so that the unit never comes in direct contact with the skin.

As with all equipment, be sure to follow manufacturer guidelines for maintenance. These may vary widely based on the output of the light, materials used to construct it, and potential hazards caused by treating a light with a specific solution. Pre-service considerations and post-treatment protocols will need to be followed to prevent any existing conditions from worsening instead of improving.

Laser and IPL Devices

Intense pulsed light, commonly referred to as IPL, and laser devices may be used by estheticians in hair removal or photorejuvenation services (Figure 4–18a, 4–18b). One aspect of IPL and laser safety is dealing with the release of a "plume" that is generated by the device when it contacts the skin.

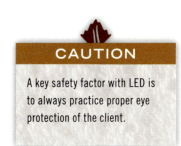

CAUTION

A key safety factor with LED is to always practice proper eye protection of the client.

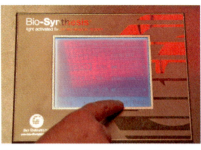

FIGURE 4–18A Free standing LED skin treatment device.

© Milady, a part of Cengage Learning. Photography by Rob Werfel.

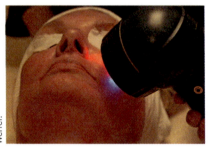

FIGURE 4–18B Hand-held LED skin treatment device.

© Milady, a part of Cengage Learning. Photography by Rob Werfel.

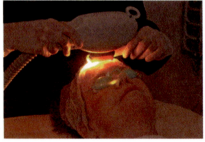

FIGURE 4–19 Proper use of an IPL device.

© Milady, a part of Cengage Learning. Photography by Rob Werfel.

For hair removal, this nearly invisible output contains noxious odors and potential biohazards. It is important to have the appropriate High-Efficiency Particulate Air (HEPA) filtration and purifying system in place to remove any microparticles of hair, skin, or smoke and the chemical compounds that are formed in the treatment process.

Client screening and pre- and post-treatment compliance are critical to minimizing overall risk. The number of legal issues with IPL and laser hair removal has grown equivalent to the number of clients seeking this service. For personal protection, every esthetician offering this type of treatment should receive complete and reliable training, maintain certifications, and ensure clients' compliance is granted for all pre- and post-treatment recommendations (Figure 4–19). Non-adherence to safety protocols can result in hyper- or hypopigmentation, burns, scars, or infections. Other common concerns are erythema and edema following IPL and laser hair removal.

IPL and laser devices are sophisticated units that require routine professional maintenance. Maintenance and service contracts are costly and may run from $5000 to $10,000 or even higher, depending on the device involved. Be sure that a service contract is negotiated at the time of purchasing your device. Considerations for a contract include parts, labor, and preventive maintenance. Annual recertification on any device is commonly required. Insurance firms may have different requirements to gain insurance coverage for IPL and laser devices. Check with your insurance agency to determine what recertification may be required.

Every manufacturer has specific protocols that must be adhered to in order for the warranty and professional liability insurance coverage to be maintained. Thorough training is required to operate IPL or laser devices safely. Any technician operating as a "solo" technician becomes, by default, the Laser Safety Officer (LSO). This position requires specific annual education in order to meet American National Standards Institute (ANSI) requirements. The ANSI standards are used as the legal benchmarks should a lawsuit be brought against a technician.

Specific considerations for IPL and laser safety include the following:

- Wipe down the unit daily.
- Wipe down the unit following each procedure.
- Properly disinfect hand-piece components after each use.
- Check lens glass and disinfect following manufacturer's directions.
- Never leave key in device.
- Never leave an active unit unattended.
- If using topical anesthetics, follow directions carefully.
- Check protective eyewear for scratches daily.
- Disinfect client eyewear after every treatment.
- Require every client to wear the correct protective eye coverings.
- Place appropriate signs outside treatment door prior to treatment.
- Carefully follow manufacturer recommendations for treatment settings.

The heads of laser and IPL units generate high levels of heat. There is always a risk of burns or triggering of flammable ingredients. Improper use may result in combustion or fire. Follow manufacturer directions for disinfection carefully to protect both the client and the technician. Some of these heads are single-use to reduce the risk of cross contamination. If a device does not have disposable heads, seek training in how to disinfect heads that will be reused.

Ultraviolet Sanitizer

Ultraviolet light has been demonstrated to be an effective method for disinfecting liquids such as water in swimming pools. It is frequently used for this in municipal water supplies. For tools and implements, however, UV sanitizing equipment follows the definition of sanitizing by reducing germs. Such equipment is not classified as a disinfecting agent by OSHA or the CDC. Check with your state regulatory agency to determine if it is considered acceptable for you to use.

Glass Bead Sterilizer

Although marketed under the name of glass bead sterilizer, this type of unit is not approved as a "sterilizer" unit. Though it may destroy many forms of living organisms, it is not effective at killing spores. This type of unit was popular 20 years ago with the dental profession but has since been eliminated because it does not meet CDC requirements for sterilization. If an esthetician has one, it can be used following other disinfection processes as an add-on precaution, but it is not a replacement for an autoclave or other high-level disinfection that may be required by states.

If a glass bead unit is used, follow the manufacturer's directions for the frequency with which beads need to be replaced and ensure that the unit is heating properly. Use care around this device, as the cup that holds the beads gets very hot and burns can result. Most of these units are not of an adequate size to hold more than the tip of an implement. The body of the implement is not exposed to any disinfecting properties, making for an insufficient result.

Autoclave

An autoclave is a device that will subject implements to high-pressure saturated steam for a specified period of time. Autoclaves are an effective method for sterilizing implements that can tolerate the heat, moisture, and pressure. Scissors, tweezers, comedone extractors, and other critical devices must be autoclaved to assure the highest level of client safety. As discussed in Chapter 2, sterilization can only be achieved when specific standards are met and when indicators, integrators, and spore testing are routinely performed. The autoclave itself must also be cleaned and maintained to ensure effectiveness. Follow the manufacturer's directions for autoclave cleaning. Autoclave units are heavy, so make sure the cleaning process is done with extra precaution to avoid the risk of personal injury.

The sterilizing chamber of an autoclave should be cleaned on a weekly basis. This is carried out by emptying the reservoir and thoroughly cleaning the inside of the chamber with a mild soap and distilled water. No abrasives or bleach should be used. Completely rinse with distilled water and then refill the reservoir. The rubber door gasket should be wiped down daily, inspected for cracks, and replaced as necessary. On a monthly basis, the autoclave should be flushed using the manufacturer recommended sterilizing cleaner.

Basic autoclave cleaning steps include:

1. Carefully move the autoclave to the edge of a sink.
2. Position the drain on the bottom of the autoclave so that it will drain into the sink.
3. Loosen the petcock screw on the bottom of the unit and allow the water to drain into the sink.
4. Close the petcock and secure the autoclave on the counter.
5. Pour autoclave cleaner that has been premixed with distilled water according to manufacturer directions into the holding tank.
6. Run a cycle following manufacturer's directions but do not sterilize any implements on this run.
7. Drain any remaining water/cleaner blend from the autoclave holding tank into the sink, then close petcock and refill the tank with fresh distilled water.
8. Run 2 (two) cycles to rinse the autoclave and reservoir tank.
9. Allow the unit to cool, then drain the tank again. Remove internal trays and wipe down the inside of the chamber, being careful of the heating element if exposed.
10. Refill the reservoir with distilled water to prepare it for the next load of items to be sterilized.

Periodically, the autoclave should be inspected by a trained service person to check the rubber grommets and components. This will confirm the reliability of the equipment and ensure that mechanical components are operating safely. Service personnel can be located through a medical or dental equipment maintenance supply.

Other Devices

Each year, new devices are introduced and promoted to the professional esthetic market. It is important that basic safety factors are considered prior to investing in any new equipment. Begin by checking whether the equipment meets the standards outlined on the National Coalition of Estheticians, Manufacturers/Distributors and Associations (NCEA) equipment evaluation form. The unit must be disinfectable so that there is no risk of cross-contamination from client to client. The technician must have adequate training in every type of equipment use offered as a treatment to ensure client safety and adherence to national safety and infection-control standards.

To adhere to these guidelines, check with each manufacturer as to the appropriate solutions for obtaining proper disinfection. It is essential to understand which infection-control processes and procedures can be implemented to maximize client and technician comfort and safety without causing damage to the equipment. Always observe the device and consider what components are touched during a treatment and how those components can be disinfected. Consider how those components can be sterilized before coming in contact with the next client. Research any special storage requirement for the unit, as well as the cost efficiency of replacement parts. With any equipment, a knowledgeable investment will lead to safer practices and more reliable results.

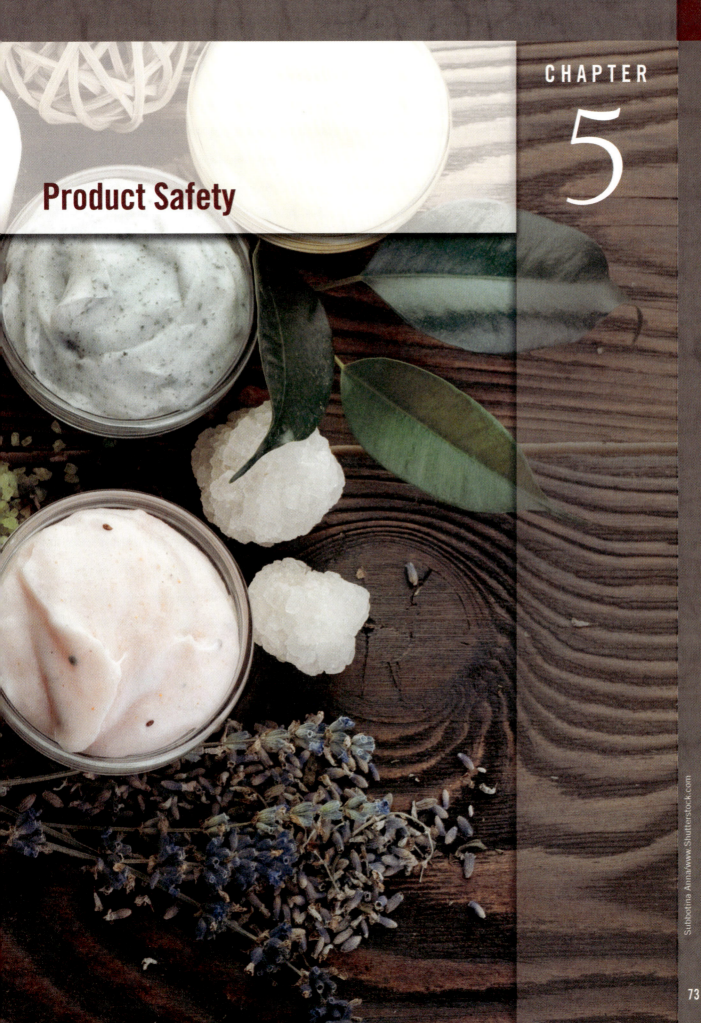

Product Safety

INTRODUCTION

Esthetic products are intended to improve and maintain professional treatments performed on the skin. The correct and appropriate selection, care, and use of products are equal in importance to the proper selection care and use of equipment. In order to offer the optimal amount of quality treatments, an esthetician must select the best product to use based on the needs of the client, the product ingredients, and manufacturer recommendations. Ingredient knowledge is crucial to avoid skin irritations and allergic reactions. Following protocols for product use can minimize the risk of any negative results. Every manufacturer has a unique formula developed in a specific manner. This allows for a wide variety of product types available, and each professional should learn what makes each formula behave differently and follow the unique directions of the manufacturer.

FOLLOW MANUFACTURER GUIDELINES

FYI

With many types of peels available, you may have been trained in one AHA, BHA, or enzyme, but do not assume that every product out there with the same name will be the same in formula and usage. Seek training from the manufacturer in the product brand you will be using and follow its guidelines.

Manufacturers provide specific guidelines for their products and equipment. This information should include a list of cautions and contraindications that cover both medical conditions and allergies to be aware of. This information will be based from the ingredients in the product and the interactions with the skin. For example, packaging for a product that contains almond oil may state that clients who have nut allergies are considered to be contraindicated. Another product may caution that allergic reactions may be triggered in people who are allergic to yeast, bees, or seaweed. As trends move to more botanically based products, there may be more client sensitivities due to common plant allergies. When selecting products for a client, either for home care or for treatment room use, we need to be aware of general health, skin issues, allergies, and any medications that could have an impact.

MSDS

Occupational Safety and Health Administration (OSHA) mandates that the clinic have a Material Safety Data Sheet (MSDS) on file for all products used. The MSDS provides all pertinent and necessary product information, including hazardous ingredients, physical and chemical properties, health hazard data, and precautions for safe use. This can be especially helpful in the event of a client reaction. If necessary, you may easily copy the MSDS and provide it to the medical practitioner so he or she can offer the best course of treatment. Any time you are purchasing a new product line, always request MSDS forms from the manufacturer and create an organized in-clinic file for quick access (Figure 5–1). An easy and popular method is using a three-ring binder with dividers based on manufacturer or product type, which allow for speedy access. Ensure that all staff are trained on the location of the MSDS binder; an additional copy may need to be made available in a larger facility. MSDS should also be on file for all types of cleaning agents or other chemicals used in the facility.

Material Safety Data Sheet (MSDS)

Section I

Product Name or Number	Emergency Telephone No.
Manufacturer's Name	Manufacturer's D-U-N-5 No.
Address (Number, Street, City, State, Zip)	
Hazardous Materials Description and Proper Shipping Name (49.CFR 172.101)	Hazardous Class (49.CFR 172.101)
Chemical Family	Formula

Section II — Ingredients (list all ingredients)   CASE REGISTRY NO.   %

Section III — Physical Data

Boiling Point (F) (C)		Specific Gravity (H20 = 1)		
Vapor Pressure (mm Hg) _____		Percent Volatile by Volume (%)		
(psl) _____				
Vapor Density (Air = 1)		Evaporation Rate (= 1)		
Solubility in Water		pH =		
Appearance and Odor		Is material: Liquid Solid Gas Paste Powder		

Section IV — Fire & Explosion Hazard Data

Flash Point (method used)	Flammable Limits	LEL	UEL
( )			
( )			
Extinguishing Media			
Special Fire Fighting Procedures			
Unusual Fire and Explosion Hazards			

FIGURE 5–1 An MSDS form containing pertinent and necessary information about a product is available from the manufacturer.

Shelf Life

A "shelf life" is the length of time a product may be stored before it begins to lose its freshness or effectiveness. All products have a manufacturer-recommended shelf life. Since this can vary from weeks to years, it is important to find out from the manufacturer what the shelf life is for each individual product and to ensure that the product has been date-stamped. Exposure to air will affect shelf life, so check with the manufacturer or product representative if packaging does not limit air exposure. The date stamp may be a batch expiration date or a manufacturing date. Some manufacturers guarantee their product for a specific amount of time from the date of purchase. In this case, the products should be marked with the date of purchase. A fine-tipped permanent marking pen simplifies this; the date should be placed on the bottom or back of container for ease of viewing. Only purchase the quantity of supplies you can use during the recommended shelf life.

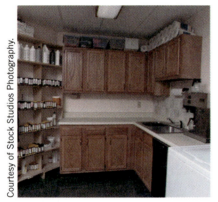

FIGURE 5–2 A proper storage area is helpful to maintain the integrity of products.

Courtesy of Stock Studios Photography.

Storage

Proper storage is also critical to maintaining the integrity of products (Figure 5–2). Avoid storing in direct sunlight, or near heat sources like radiators. Some products may require refrigeration, but most are stable at room temperature. Products that require refrigeration must be stored in a separate unit from one used for consumable items such as food or drinks. Products may separate or change consistency at very low or high temperatures. Some pure essential oils—for example, Bulgarian Rose Otto—will crystallize if kept in a very cool room. This is inherent in this oil and an indication of its purity; upon returning to room temperature, the crystals completely disappear.

Most products do not respond well to excessive heat. Items such as lipstick or wax pellets may melt if shipped in very hot weather or when stored too closely to a heat source. With wax-based products, heat generally does not affect product function but the usability of some products such lipstick can be compromised. Likewise, shipping during extremely cold conditions may also affect some products. If in doubt, check with the manufacturer for advice and policies on replacement of damaged product. Avoid performing treatments on a client using products that have been subject to temperature extremes unless this has been approved by the manufacturer.

Treatment Room Protocols

Esthetic services and product use in the treatment room is different from what may be recommended for a client to use at home. In order to have safe and effective treatment results, estheticians must choose products that will help achieve goals but not cause problematic irritation to the client's skin.

Case Study

On maturing skin, a client may use a gentle, milky cleanser at home. In the treatment room, this product is excellent for removing makeup but not for preparing the skin for exfoliation. In this circumstance, the esthetician may safely use a cleanser with deeper penetration after removing the makeup to prepare skin for the exfoliation step.

Case Study

A client with oily or acne-prone skin will probably use a clay mask at home. In the treatment room, if we have performed a stimulating treatment, we can safely use a gentle gel-based mask or a hydrating collagen fiber mask to calm and soothe the skin. This is safer for the client than using the absorbing clay mask, as it will reduce any skin irritation.

Toners are another category where we can safely use products on the client in the treatment room that may not be appropriate for them on a daily basis at home. The key is selecting the correct treatment for the client and following the manufacturer's guidelines.

Allergies

Allergies and sensitivities are a crucial area that every esthetician should be educated in. Whether performing a facial or body treatment, the technician must know specifically what substances may provoke a reaction in a client and be prepared to deal with any type of allergic response. All intake forms should include a detailed section on allergies. It is also important to find out what sort of response a client has to an allergen: is it localized and only showing redness, or systemic and causing negative health effects? For a client with numerous allergies or extreme reactions, consider asking if the client has ever had an anaphylactic response and whether he or she carries an EpiPen to deal with the allergy.

Specific Allergic Responses

As mentioned previously, many people have allergies or are sensitive to plant pollens or specific foods. Estheticians have the responsibility to seek out this information and avoid products with these allergens in them. Allergies can be congenital or develop with repeated use or exposure to an agent. This does not mean that the agent is bad for everyone; it simply means that an individual has developed a sensitivity to that specific agent. The agent may be one specific

CAUTION

Never spray toners into the air that contain astringents or SD alcohol in them. When sprayed into the air, these can cause respiratory irritation and trigger a cough reflex. Instead, apply the product to a cotton or gauze pad and then wipe the skin with it.

CAUTION

Avoid contamination of products when removing them from the original container. Never use your hands to dip into a container and always use a disposable spatula or wooden tongue blade.

FYI

One example of allergic reactions due to exposure comes with the use of haircolor products. Women may color their hair for many years without any problems and then suddenly have a mild or severe reaction to the coloring agent. This type of allergic reaction occurs when a person becomes sensitized to a product ingredient. Continued exposure to some agents will result in this response. In this situation, other alternatives such as different products or methods must be investigated to prevent future problems for the client. This does not mean that the coloring product used is a bad product; it is simply one that that particular person can no longer tolerate.

ingredient, plant life, a food item, pet dander, or type of fiber; some people are even sensitive to their own immune response.

Excessive application or overuse of a product can increase the risk of developing sensitivity to a product. This is termed "overexposure," and prevention is crucial by following manufacturer instructions for application methods and time limits of use. Clients may request more of a product, hoping to get a stronger response. No matter how aggressive or pleading the client gets, never fail to follow the manufacturer instructions, as this can result in a negative response or the development of a loss of tolerance for the product.

Case Study

A client entered a spa requesting to have her lashes to be tinted for her camping vacation. She encouraged the technician to apply the product more heavily so that the base of the lashes would turn out darker. Against the product instructions and her better judgment, the esthetician complied to please the client. The client returned about six weeks later for another eyelash tint. Immediately upon application of the tint product, the client reported that her eyes were watering and burning. The product was speedily removed and the area inspected. The area showed inflammation and redness. Upon being questioned about any prior similar response, the client admitted that following her last eyelash tint treatment she had ended up with an eye irritation that lasted several days. Due to the client's eagerness for more color, she has now experienced sensitivity due to overexposure that makes receiving this service in the future contraindicated.

Case Study

A client visited a spa for a body wrap. The esthetician performed a full-body seaweed wrap for her. Once the client was cocooned, the technician briefly left the room to retrieve more supplies. Upon returning, the client appeared disoriented and was having trouble speaking clearly. The esthetician immediately sought the assistance of her manager. The client's condition quickly worsened and the manager called 9-1-1. When the paramedics arrived, the client passed out and the emergency responders began medical treatment to the client, concerned about the possibility of a heart attack. In actuality, the client was suffering anaphylactic shock due to being allergic to the seaweed. The client died while in route to the hospital. Later, it was discovered that her death was due to a severe allergic reaction resulting in anaphylactic shock.

Estheticians should be on the lookout for undetected allergies. Sometimes a client may not consider an allergy to food a potential problem for their spa treatment, so they may omit information or simply forget to mention it. Remaining with a client at all times is the first step to preventing these issues. If the client becomes disoriented, complains of discomfort, or suddenly starts behaving oddly, remove any product on the skin immediately, as the client response could be an allergic reaction. Never delay taking action if an allergy may be possible or if you have any doubt or concern. In case of any doubt, properly remove the product from the skin. Be sure to implement an internal alert to obtain support, and call for medical help if the client still seems disoriented. Protocols for doing this will be discussed in the chapter on handling emergency and non-emergency situations.

Patch Testing

If there is ever a question about the suitability of a product or ingredient for a client, taking the time to complete a patch test is crucial to a favorable outcome. Any skin can be reactive, and it is important to patch-test clients if sensitivity is suspected or if the manufacturer recommends patch testing in its directions for use (Figure 5–3).

A patch or skin response test may be done on the inside of the elbow or on the back. Avoid testing behind the ear, as this is where fragrance is commonly placed and an interaction could occur. Begin by cleansing the test area and apply a small amount of the product in question. Watch closely for any redness or response. A patch test may be done a little differently for products that are intended for short- or long-term contact with the skin. Reactions may occur immediately or over a prolonged period of time; possible reactions include itching, burning, inflammation, or irritation of the skin.

Provided here is the series of steps to be taken when completing a patch or skin response test.

1. If the product to be tested is normally applied and then removed, such as an acid, complete on a test area according to manufacturer directions. Following removal of the product, examine the area for signs of irritation or inflammation. Wait 48–72 hours and recheck the condition of the skin in the test area. If the skin appears to be in a normal state, you may proceed with the use of the product.
2. If the product to be tested is one that will remain on the skin, apply the product and then cover with a labeled bandage and check in 48–72 hours. The area should be kept dry. If the area becomes inflamed or irritated, advise the client to remove the product immediately and contact you. The product should not be used on this client. If there is no sign of irritation and the skin appears normal, then it is likely safe to proceed with application of that product.

Enzymes

Enzymes destroy the keratin in dead surface cells and are referred to as peels, masks, or treatments. Prior to performing enzyme treatments, seek proper training for mixing, application, and removal of any enzyme treatment.

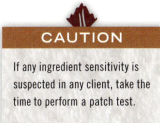

CAUTION

If any ingredient sensitivity is suspected in any client, take the time to perform a patch test.

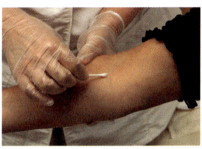

© Milady, a part of Cengage Learning, Inc. Photography by Rob Werfel.

FIGURE 5–3 Patch testing will help determine unknown allergies.

HERE'S A TIP

When performing a longer-term patch test on a client by covering with a bandage, be aware that many bandages may cause a reaction due to latex derivatives in the adhesive. A positive reaction could actually come from the bandage and not the product being tested. The best way to avoid this confusion is to purchase bandages that are less likely to cause a reaction; they will be listed as such on the label.

Case Study

An esthetician had received brief training in the use of a particular enzyme product. After an enzyme treatment, the esthetician noticed that the client's skin was slightly dry and tight immediately following the removal of the enzyme. The technician decided to buffer the enzyme by using a peptide activator instead of the manufacturer's recommended product. While there was no harm to the client, the client did waste time and money. Adding the peptide product to the enzyme neutralized it so that no exfoliation occurred. The technician also didn't understand that the tightness immediately following the enzyme was normal and even desirable. The skin would be rehydrated during subsequent steps of the treatment.

Read product information thoroughly prior to use to be informed of concerns that may occur during each portion of a treatment. Always follow manufacturer's mixing directions, and if concerned about the way a product is behaving, ask the representative for clarification. Each enzyme is made with its own unique formula, and the manufacturer may have options for making it a gentler process or enhancing its activity.

Acids

The use of different types of acids is common practice in the treatment room. Safety and success depend on adequate training and adherence to the manufacturer's guidelines. If a technician has had training using AHAs (alpha hydroxy acids) with a pH of 3.0 or higher and then attempts to use a low-pH product, such as a product with a pH of 1.7, in the manner that they were trained, the client could easily be burned. This type of burn may result in permanent scar tissue. It is critical for the technician to have proper training in the product to be used and to learn all the parameters of each product.

Many clients and even some estheticians may feel that if minimal use delivers a good result, the additional product application or extended contact time will offer a better result. This is not the case with many products, especially acids, and can result in a negative reaction. A client may have irritated skin or subclinical inflammation that cannot be seen but manifests itself in skin sensitivity. Not all problems are easily visible, and the simple fact that redness is not observed does not mean that the skin is not recovering from irritation. Problems can be avoided by following manufacturer protocols for proper treatment selection and spacing of treatments. Fine, thin, and dry skins cannot tolerate the same level of acid use as thicker, oilier skins. While clients may request more frequent or stronger treatments, it is a sign of our professionalism and knowledge that we educate them and adhere to manufacturer protocols.

It is recommended that you never perform an acid peel treatment on a new client. A technician must see how a client's skin responds to other products before he or she can safely perform an aggressive treatment. Clients have falsely reported that they have had peels in the past, and have even been known to withhold information that was critical to safe treatment because of their own desire to receive a treatment. Acceding to client demands in these situations will increase the risk that a client will present a reaction, because the esthetician followed client requests instead of manufacturer guidelines.

Fitzpatrick Types

No acid treatment should be attempted without carefully identifying the Fitzpatrick level of the client (Figure 5–4). The Fitzpatrick level will indicate how quickly or slowly the client's skin will respond to UVA radiation and is also a key indicator for the risk of hyperpigmentation following an acid treatment.

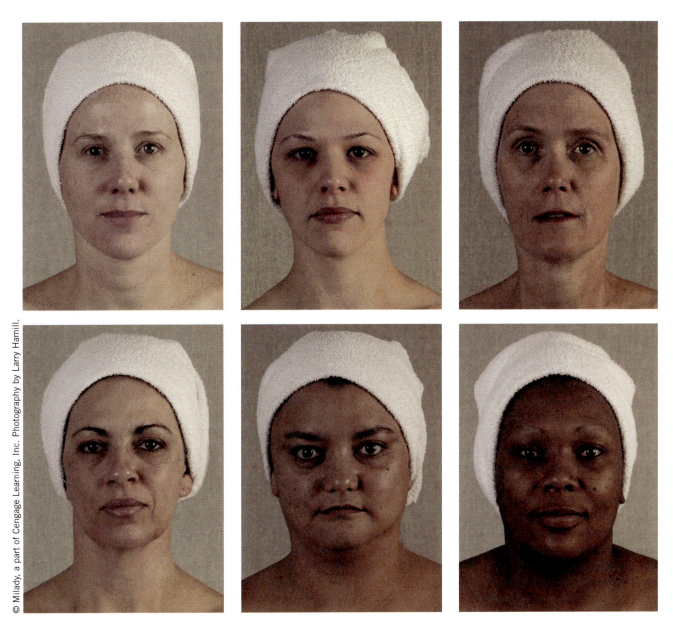

FIGURE 5–4 The Fitzpatrick Scale is used to measure the skin type's ability to tolerate sun exposure.

© Milady, a part of Cengage Learning, Inc. Photography by Larry Hamill.

Ethnic skins will have more active melanocytes than Caucasian skin types. The darker the skin tone, the higher the risk that the skin will respond to trauma by displaying post-inflammatory hyperpigmentation. This adverse reaction can take several months to two years to resolve and should be avoided. Unfortunately, these are also the clients most likely to come to the clinic seeking assistance with their hyperpigmentation. Clients may visit an esthetician requesting peels to make the dark spots go away. These treatments, however, commonly make the pigmentation more pronounced.

To safely treat hyperpigmentation, first have the client incorporate daily use of SPF (sun protection factor) cream and a lightening agent into the home-care regimen. If clients prefer not to adhere to this, they are not good candidates for a peel. Following proper home-care preparation prior to a peel treatment,

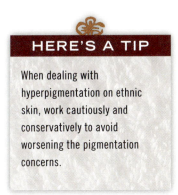

HERE'S A TIP

When dealing with hyperpigmentation on ethnic skin, work cautiously and conservatively to avoid worsening the pigmentation concerns.

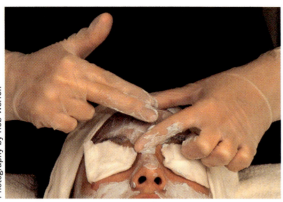

FIGURE 5-5 Always make efforts to protect the eye area when performing treatments.

select an AHA with a larger molecule size, such as a lactic or malic acid. Also, avoid products with a lower pH, as they can be more irritating and heighten the risk of hyperpigmentation. Rather than performing a standard series of peels, as would be done on a lighter skin, alternate the peel with an enzyme treatment. This will allow you to slowly coax the skin lighter to avoid adverse results.

Application Techniques

Proper product application is critical to client safety. Many products may cause problems if contact is made with the eye area or the inside of the nostrils, or if the product enters the mouth area. Correct and consistent application of an acid is a necessary safe practice. Always protect the eyes of the client with cotton pads so that any accidental drips will be absorbed by the cotton and not be allowed to enter the eye area (Figure 5–5). Many manufacturers recommend using a tiny amount of petroleum jelly under the eyes, at the base of the nose, and on the lips prior to application of an acid. If the client is prone to herpes simplex and is not on an antiviral medication, avoid the upper lip when working in close proximity to either lip. Acid treatments can trigger a herpetic breakout, so be certain to protect this area with petroleum jelly to prevent the acid from spreading here.

Never leave the room when a client has an acid applied on the skin. The client may become anxious or uncomfortable due to the sensation, or may possibly develop a negative reaction. It is critical that the esthetician be present to monitor the client and adjust the treatment if necessary. Prior to beginning the treatment, technicians should prepare by having a basin of cool water within reach for quick rinsing of the skin and having all supplies within easy reach.

Be familiar with the consistency of the product you are using. Some products have thickening agents to allow for more control during application. Other acid products have a thin, watery consistency and tend to run. Make sure the applicator tool is used properly and does not allow for any dripping. Never allow an acid to have thicker areas or puddle on the skin during application. Any uneven application of acid will result in some areas of the skin being more deeply exfoliated. Any skin area receiving excessively deep exfoliation may become an irritated or wounded spot, which could then be subject to infection, post-inflammatory hyperpigmentation, or scarring.

When removing the acid, rinse thoroughly and then rinse again. Communicate by asking for feedback from the client such as, "Do you still feel any tingling, itching, or stinging?" Requesting client feedback and explaining the importance of proper rinsing is the safest, most reliable protocol.

Some products are blended peels. These product types contain an exfoliating agent such as glycolic, lactic, salicylic, or another acid. This form of exfoliating agent is buffered and neutralized by skin oils and other ingredients incorporated into these products. These buffering and neutralizing agents mean that this unique product is left on the skin rather than removed. Estheticians must follow manufacturer guidelines for use with these products and NEVER use these techniques with other brands, as a burn to the client could occur.

Combining Treatments

Some technicians have attempted to combine mechanical exfoliation before or after acid therapy. This should only be done if it is recommended by the manufacturer. If the manufacturer cautions against this, never attempt to perform this combination of treatments.

Case Study

Some estheticians in a sunny climate desired a better result for their clients with sun-damaged skin. They decided on a course of treatment combining acid treatments with microdermabrasion. The clients quickly began complaining that their home-care products were irritating their skin, even though they had never had this problem in the past. The clients were not informed to limit their sun exposure. If clients choose to have regular sun exposure and do not consistently use SPF creams, it is unsafe to perform acid treatments on them. The clients may suffer from a sunburn or hyperpigmentation. Sun exposure is contraindicated following acid treatments. Provide every client with written guidelines for home care and sun exposure following the treatment. Require clients to sign an informed consent indicating that the guidelines have been explained to them and that they understand and agree to follow them. Always avoid unsafe practices and take all measures to prevent problems.

An esthetician may sincerely aspire to generate services and increase revenue. If manufacturer guidelines are not properly followed, there is a short-term risk of skin reactions and the long-term risk of accelerated aging. If the client still requests more than you can safely offer, refer the client to a physician rather than practicing risky treatments.

Other aggressive treatments, such as waxing, should never be combined with any acid treatment. Some estheticians and clients may claim never to have had a problem with this combination of treatments, but this decision can turn disastrous even in the hands of the experienced professional.

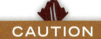

CAUTION

Never offer a wax treatment and perform any exfoliation or acid treatment over the same area on the same day.

Alpha Hydroxy Acids

When working with products containing alpha hydroxy acids (AHAs), there are some specific conditions that must be determined. Alpha hydroxy acids are naturally occurring mild acids that are sold in a variety of formulas, concentrations, and pH levels. Technicians must be aware of any state guidelines that restrict their usage. AHAs are placed on the skin, timed, and then removed to stop their action. Hyperpigmentation may occur if an accurate Fitzpatrick scale analysis is not performed.

It is crucial to know both the concentration (percentage) of an AHA and its pH factor. This particular combination indicates the aggressiveness of the treatment that the product offers. The level of treatment aggressiveness must be individualized based on the Fitzpatrick scale; more aggressive is not always better. Many estheticians have more than one level of AHA available so they can begin their clients at a 15 to 20 percent concentration before adjusting to a higher level. Other technicians prefer to use formulas that have soothing properties incorporated to minimize the risk of skin reactions. The professional goal is to improve

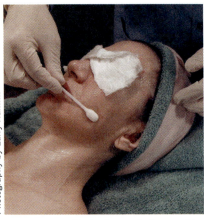

© Milady, a part of Cengage Learning, Inc.
Photography by Larry Hamill.

FIGURE 5-6 Product manufacturers will advise the best application method for peel treatments.

the appearance of the skin without triggering downtime or damage to the epidermis. Technicians desiring to perform more aggressive medical peels should only do so under medical supervision and with proper insurance coverage.

Always perform every treatment as if it is the first the client is to experience (Figure 5–6). Some clients may do well for several AHA treatments and then have a different response. This may be due to thinning of the skin or changes in health status or client home care. Stay with the client and observe and respond accordingly.

Beta Hydroxy Acids

Beta hydroxy acids (BHAs) are most commonly those that have a salicylic or citrus base. These types of products have been safely used in the treatment room for over 50 years. One advantage of BHAs is the benefits of self-timing and self-neutralizing. Once moisture has evaporated and the product is dry, the action stops. Using a fan to temper the sting of salicylic acid accelerates the drying and thereby reduces the activity. BHA should not be used on any client with salicylic allergies. Salicylic processes differently from the AHAs. It is actually metabolized through the body and removed via the excretory system. For this reason, it should be avoided with clients who are pregnant or nursing.

BHAs should never be applied to the full body, as this could result in salicylic poisoning, which can have serious, even fatal, effects. Limit use only to the face, décolleté, or upper back at one time. Body treatments are more safely done with an AHA product.

BHA products are oil-loving and can penetrate not only through the epidermis but through the oil glands, resulting in the breaking up of blocked follicles. This makes BHA treatments preferable for acneic clients. These are often available in a 12 to 25 percent concentration. To minimize irritation, start the client on a low concentration and only progress to the higher level if results are not achieved. Follow manufacturer guidelines for timing of treatments and product protocols.

Jessner's Formulations

There are numerous acids sold under the name of Jessner's or modified Jessner's. These product types have similar but not identical formulas, which causes great confusion and risk for the client. It is crucial to get complete information on any Jessner's formula being considered for use. Classical Jessner's formulations are 14 percent salicylic, 14 percent lactic, and 14 percent resorcinol in an ethanol base. The ethanol base, ethyl alcohol, acts as a disinfectant and preservative. When applied to the skin, the ethanol evaporates very quickly, pushing the formula into the skin. Modified Jessner's formulas may be weaker or stronger than the true Jessner's and may have different ingredients involved. These can greatly impact the anticipated result.

Some Jessner's product types come in a hydro-alcohol base, which means that water, and not ethyl alcohol, is used as a diluting agent. The product application may therefore be quite different. Follow manufacturer's guidelines and do not attempt to use one set of guidelines for all formulas.

CAUTION

It is important to know the base of a Jessner's solution as well as its percentages. Each one behaves differently. To prevent complications, always adhere to manufacturer's directions.

In some states, Jessner's formulation treatments are within the scope of practice for estheticians to use; in others, they are not. Technicians must be aware of their individual state guidelines and whether the state guidelines are based on concentrations or buffering and non-buffering formulas. In most states, the technician is responsible for obtaining proper training before administering any product to the client's skin and working within the scope of practice. Failure to do so could result in loss of a technician's professional license. Finding and understanding the regulations can sometimes require research and investigation.

Another example of this is that classical Jessner's solutions are applied in not more than one to two coats for esthetic use and three to five coats for use by physicians. Some companies offer a modified formula for purchase that calls for as many six to seven coats. If an esthetician who had been trained in this diluted formula later switched brands, there could be serious risk of injury for the client. We must KNOW our product and not make assumptions based on the product name.

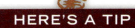

HERE'S A TIP

It is the responsibility of all estheticians to research their products, to make sure that those products are within their scope of practice to use, and to be thoroughly trained in the use of the products.

Trichloracetic Acid

Trichloracetic acid (TCA) is considered more than a superficial peel by most experts. It is less predictable and carries a higher risk factor for consequences, side effects, and complications. Outbreaks of impetigo have been known to result from TCA treatments. This is a protocol best done under physician supervision. Estheticians using this treatment in states where it is allowed must have product-specific training, and should make sure their insurance covers this peel and prepare a list of medical professionals to back them up if an incident occurs.

Essential Oils and Botanicals

Essential oils can be a fabulous tool for every esthetician by providing numerous benefits (Figure 5–7). Unfortunately, these items are also a potential allergen because they are the

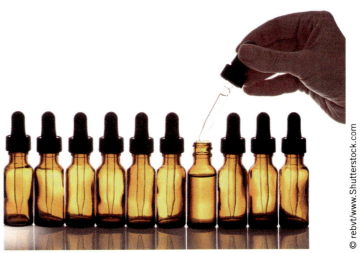

FIGURE 5–7 Essential oils are frequently used in esthetic treatments and products.

© rebvt/www.Shutterstock.com

most powerful part of the plant. For an esthetician wanting to use essential oils in the treatment room, specialized training is mandatory. Begin with the basics; there is much to learn about essential oils and it can take quite some time to master the topic due to the complex nature of the plant attributes and the many ways they can affect the body. Not only can essential oils cause skin reactions, the wrong oil on the wrong client can have a negative impact on the client's health or cause a detoxification that the client could interpret as negative. Generally speaking, if the use of the essential oils is discontinued, any irritation will be alleviated. Most negative concerns result from a technician not following correct formulation protocols or attempting to work with an unfamiliar essential oil. It is critical to learn the cautions and contraindications for essential oils and safe ways to incorporate them. Those oils that are photosensitizing should be used with caution in sunny climates and not be applied to a client's skin prior to sun exposure.

Common photosensitizing oils are listed for you here:

- Bergamot
- Lemon
- Lime
- Bitter orange
- Angelica

Always practice extreme care when dealing with clients with existing health issues, as their response to oils could be stronger and unpredictable. Certain health issues to be aware of prior to using essential oils include:

- Cancer
- HIV
- Pregnancy
- High or low blood pressure
- Emotional instability

The following oils are potential skin irritants; use only blended and in low concentrations. Another alternative might be to use them indirectly, such as in a diffuser.

- Evergreen oils such as cypress, pine, and spruce
- Citrus oils such as grapefruit, lemon, and orange
- Frankincense
- Lemon verbena
- Melissa
- Lemongrass
- Citronella
- Eucalyptus citriodora
- Oregano
- Thyme thymol
- Savory
- Cinnamon
- Clove

Phenylpropane derivatives, including anise seed, basil, fennel, nutmeg, and tarragon, are toxic to the nervous system in very high doses and so should only be included in low concentrations.

CAUTION

When performing treatments on pregnant clients, avoid using any form of ketone oils, as they can be neurotoxic and abortive. These include mugwort, thuja, and pennyroyal.

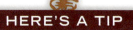

HERE'S A TIP

Safe concentrations of essential oils for estheticians are generally considered to be 0.5 to 2.5 percent. For information on creating an essential oil blend, consult the Essential Oil chapter in *Milady Standard Esthetics: Advanced* or Jimm Harrison's *Aromatherapy: Therapeutic Use of Essential Oils for Esthetics* (Cengage Learning, 2008).

One safe way to start with essential oils is to add a few drops of oil, either a single-note oil or a manufacturer's pre-mixed blend, to the water in which towels are to be dipped before placing them in the towel cabbie. Only trace amounts of the oil will remain on the towel and they will give a light and pleasant aroma to the room. The manufacturer blends are nice, as you can be assured the ingredients are balanced to work together. When mixing essential oils, the result is synergistic, and the action of the blend will be greater than the action that each oil would individually produce.

During seasonal changes, when bacteria and viruses cause numerous illnesses, the presence of the oil can be a bonus disinfectant. A small amount may be placed in a diffuser for a holistic approach to client health. All essential oils have some antibacterial, antifungal, antiviral, and antiseptic properties, but some specific oils are more commonly used for this purpose.

Oils that are commonly used for benefits of controlling environmental microbes and for the enhancement of respiratory comfort include the following:

- Eucalyptus
- Tea tree
- Pine
- Thyme
- Pre-blended product such as one for respiration

When using essential oils in the treatment room, follow recommended handling safety precautions. Never place any essential oils directly on a client or into a steamer, which could result in a topical or systemic reaction. Instead, utilize a diffusion method such as placing oils in an electric or ceramic diffuser.

Basic guidelines for use of essential oils are provided here:

- Unless specifically directed by the manufacturer, do not apply essential oils directly to the skin, sometimes called "neat." Always dilute into carrier oil.
- Avoid getting essential oils near the eyes, nose, mouth, or ears.
- Do not ingest essential oils.
- Essential oils are flammable; keep them away from light bulbs, flame, and other volatile sources.
- Patch-test before incorporating into client products using a 2 percent solution in carrier oil.
- Store tightly capped away from light and heat.
- Keep out of the reach of children and pets.
- Do not make assumptions about the properties of an essential oil.
- Follow all manufacturer directions.

Botanicals are the plants, herbs, flowers, roots, and bark from which essential oils are derived. The plants themselves are commonly used in skin care for their various properties. Botanicals are considered safer than essential oils because they are not as concentrated. Due to possible environmental contaminants and product liability issues, estheticians should obtain their botanicals from reliable manufacturers rather than from their own gardens. Every batch of botanicals processed commercially is tested to assure that the desired components are present in the expected ranges. Botanical manufacturers use these test results to select the ingredients they will use in the product preparation. Using professional products is a key to client safety. Clients can be equally or even more reactive to botanicals than to essential oils, so always adhere to safety practices (Harrison, 2008).

Mixing Products

This refers to the process of mixing together products from various manufacturers. This is an unsafe practice. No manufacturer will stand behind its product if the product has been altered. Insurance providers commonly exclude the practice of mixing products beyond the scope of manufacturer directions from their coverage. Estheticians who wish to offer treatments performed with self-formulated products will need to obtain special insurance coverage.

The risk is that ingredients from two different formulators, or even two products from the same manufacturer that are not designed to work together, could be incompatible or trigger an unexpected response when placed on a client's skin. Always keep in mind that products used separately with positive results may deliver a completely different result when used together. Even if you conduct personal experiments that appear to work with acceptable results, the experimental treatment may not cause a positive reaction for your client.

Body Treatment Products

Body treatment products have the added concern that they are applied over the full body rather than on a limited area. This increased coverage and exposure ultimately increases the chances of a reaction to the product applied. This can have disastrous results. Varying degrees of skin thickness may lead to faster absorption in some areas with the use of topically applied products. This also means that we must know what ingredients these products contain and their contraindications.

Highly stimulating products should be used with caution when treating the full body; this product type may have a stronger impact on underlying medical conditions, including elevated blood pressure. Many clients take numerous medications or have special dietary needs that may affect a treatment and make a desired treatment contraindicated. It is the esthetician's responsibility to address this concern and redirect the client to a safer treatment.

Heat and occlusion, such as that created by a wrap or the incorporation of stones, also intensify the treatment and can also impact those with blood pressure or heart issues. Cold temperatures can also have a powerful effect on the body, whether they come from applying cold products to the skin, from using cold towels, or from the client experiencing a sudden temperature drop during product removal. Protocols must be established to minimize the risk of too-sudden increases or decreases in client body temperature. This is a health concern as well as a consideration for client comfort.

Waxing, Sugaring, and Paraffin

Wax and sugaring products are mired in controversy because of concerns about client safety and infection control. Professional estheticians must keep up to date

FYI

Always follow manufacturer guidelines for the use and mixing of products; unsafe practices can be dangerous and are unprofessional.

CAUTION

Always follow manufacturer directions for body treatments. This should include a thorough check of the skin for any abrasions and a product check for appropriate temperature before applying it to the client's skin.

on the most recent and stringent guidelines that follow CDC standards to prevent the spread of disease. When performing hair removal, exfoliation occurs and there is always a risk of removing more skin layers than is desirable. If the skin appears shiny, the stratum corneum layer of the skin has been removed and the client is now at risk for pathogens entering their skin. As we noted in the Infections Control chapter, the nose, underarm, and groin are all common areas for higher levels of staph. Estheticians cannot afford to take the risk that a client requesting a Brazilian waxing service will transmit germs to the subsequent eyebrow client. It is part of your professional practices to be informed and follow all CDC guidelines, and is expected by state regulations and clients (Figure 5–8).

To protect both client and technician, adhere to the following safety guidelines for waxing or sugaring treatments.

- Always have client fill out a client intake form.
- Provide client with aftercare directions and have them sign an informed consent stating that they will follow these guidelines.
- At every appointment, update this information and check to see what health, medication, and lifestyle changes may have occurred.
- Never treat a client for whom there are contraindications.
- Tanning beds and exposure to UV should be discontinued at least 48 hours prior to waxing and not resumed for 72 hours following waxing.
- If a client is prone to skin reactions or ingrown hairs, proper home-care products should be recommended and made readily available.
- Ensure that you have an appropriate product for the area to be treated.
- Clean the area to be treated before and after hair removal to minimize risk of folliculitis.
- Wear disposable gloves and replace if their barrier becomes compromised.

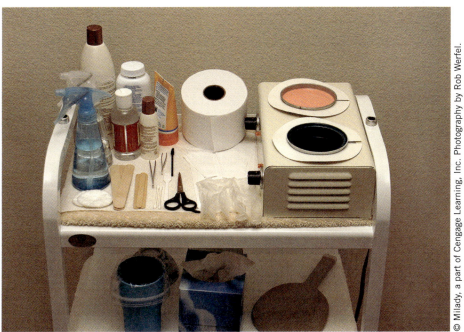

© Milady, a part of Cengage Learning, Inc. Photography by Rob Werfel.

FIGURE 5–8 Example of a clean wax cart setup.

- Use single-use disposable wax applicators.
- Never double-dip an applicator tool into any container.
- Avoid roll-on applicators unless the manufacturer can provide written documentation that there is no backflow into the cartridge. Changing a cartridge roller or top does not eliminate microbes and dead skin being carried from the skin back into the cartridge as the roller turns. Roll-on units should be for home hair removal maintenance.
- When working with the sugar ball method, never place used sugar back into the original container, and properly dispose of used product. Also change gloves prior to dipping back into the heater to collect fresh sugar.
- Always test the temperature of the wax before applying to the client's skin and make sure the comfort level of the client is communicated.
- Following the completion of the service, properly sanitize any containers that may have been handled during the procedure.
- Properly dispose of tools that cannot be disinfected.
- Clean, disinfect, and sterilize any implements that are non-disposable following standard precaution guidelines.

HERE'S A TIP

Perform a self-evaluation of your hair removal practices and the maintenance of the area following a treatment; then consider whether you would be willing to be your next client.

Wax and sugar products are temperature-sensitive. If this type of product is not warm enough, it will drag on the skin and not remove the hair, resulting in discomfort instead. If the heater is set too hot, the product can change color, texture, and consistency, resulting in diminished hair removal. Overheated products may also burn the client during application. If you are using a wax that comes in pellets and they have become stuck together during shipping or storage, place the bag in a tray to avoid scattering pellets and carefully use a rubber mallet to break them apart. Some wax comes in blocks that may need to be broken to fit in a heating unit. This should be done in a manner to prevent splattering wax particles and followed by a thorough cleanup.

Unless the heating unit specifically says to place the product directly into it, always place the wax or sugar in the recommended holder, which is held in the heater. This prevents the product from being in too close contact with the heating source and gives a double-boiler effect. This practice will better control the temperature of the product and also allows for switching out different hair removal products in the same heater.

Routinely use a wax removal cleaner to keep the heater, counters, and surrounding area free of product drips and smears. This should be done daily and not overlooked until it is convenient. Accumulation of product is unsanitary and unsafe. Keep all hair removal units and products covered when not in use so that airborne particulates cannot settle on sticky surfaces. Be aware that a hair removal unit that utilizes a lid or cover may cause the temperature to be higher than expected due to a lesser degree of heat being released. If the hair removal unit is used in an area where hair services are offered, efforts should be made to prevent hair from settling into the product. Trimmed hair and salon products can easily float into open containers. Preventing cross-contamination is critical for the products in the hair removal process.

Paraffin treatments offer many benefits for the skin as well as being a soothing and therapeutic treatment. The paraffin should be heated to a temperature of 126 to 134 degrees Fahrenheit. Be prepared in advance, as it will take 8 to 10 hours for a large-capacity heater to melt the paraffin. Paraffin heaters that are used often can be tested on a monthly basis to assure the thermostat is functioning properly; refer to the equipment manual for the best method of completing this.

Maintenance of a paraffin heater includes cleaning the unit once a month and wiping the exterior following each use. Provided for you are the steps for proper paraffin tank cleaning:

- Place a long piece of gauze into the melted paraffin, ensuring that it touches the bottom and sides of the tub with the ends hanging over the edge for easy grasping.
- Turn off the unit.
- Once the unit has cooled and the paraffin solidified, lift the gauze, removing the paraffin with it.
- Clean and then disinfect the interior of the tub with a disinfectant.
- Replace the paraffin and turn the unit back on.

Cross-contamination is a concern when using a paraffin heater; however, be informed that if proper disinfection protocols are followed, bacteria and fungi will not live in paraffin. Paraffin does not contain any oxygen or water as a food source for these organisms. Proper safe use of a paraffin heater includes always cleaning the hands or feet with antimicrobial soap or waterless gel prior to dipping; do not dip any body part that has a skin abrasion or open cut. Never place used paraffin back into the heater and always keep a lid covering the equipment when not in use (Schmaling, 2009).

Regardless of the product to be used or the area of the body it is to be used on, it is imperative that the technician have enough information about both the product and the client to ensure a positive result. Always use every product in strict accordance with manufacturer guidelines. If an esthetician chooses to not follow the manufacturer's recommended directions for use, there is an extremely high risk of client injury or dissatisfaction. Unsafe practices are never a wise decision and may lead to loss of insurance coverage and/or licensure.

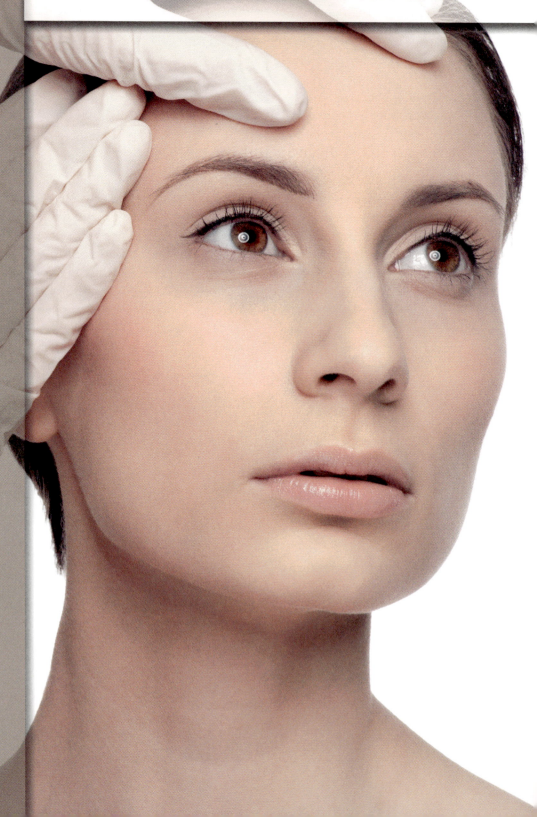

Cautions and Contraindications

INTRODUCTION

Clients will visit an esthetician for many reasons. They may desire to relax and relieve stress, to be pampered, or to preserve or improve the appearance of their skin. Clients commonly seek assistance with blackheads, dull skin, acne, Rosacea, aging skin, brown spots, oily skin, dry skin, removal of unwanted hair, or assistance in the selection or application of cosmetic products. A professional esthetician must sort through available options and match the best treatment, based not only their indications for a procedure but on any cautionary conditions that exist. Health issues such as pregnancy, diabetes, medications, and lifestyle are all examples of things estheticians must take into consideration. Proper use of the client intake form will assist in gathering information about cautions and contraindications.

CONDITIONS AND TREATMENT CHOICE

The client may exhibit conditions that provide guidance in the proper selection of treatment and the products to be used. Such conditions may be long-term and consistent, or they may alter with each visit. The esthetician must monitor all conditions on every visit to assure the best treatment practice is offered. Just because a treatment worked well for a client last time does not necessarily make it the perfect choice for every visit. A common example of this is an increase in stress level and its impact on the skin or even personal health conditions.

Stress

Busy lifestyles, family and work situations, and health concerns lead most everyone to experience stress. Suffering from stress may cause an internal cascade of events that affects every part of the human body. Some examples of stress the esthetician will be faced with include visible conditions called clinical inflammation, or things that aren't visible called subclinical inflammation. Redness, breakouts, chafed skin, and peeling are all examples of visible skin conditions that can result from stress. Non-visible impacts of excess stress may be inadequate sleep, tiredness, lack of energy, poor memory, getting sick more easily, depression, and loss of libido. Physical side effects that are visible may be weight gain or loss, nervousness, agitation, or an inability to relax. Stress often results in tension being stored in the muscular and nervous system of the body, leading to muscle aches, headaches, and a general poor feeling.

Skin treatments can certainly be beneficial to assist stressed clients in relaxing. Efforts to relieve a client's stress level begin with offering a positive impact on the senses for the most benefit. Maintaining the environment and taking care to offer a soothing, relaxing ambiance will generate feelings of restfulness and relaxation (Figure 6–1).

Suggestions for proper ambiance should be based on the senses and include:

- Vision—What the client sees from the moment he or she enters, and the level of lighting and its variations before, during and after the treatment; wall colors and decor as well as general cleanliness.

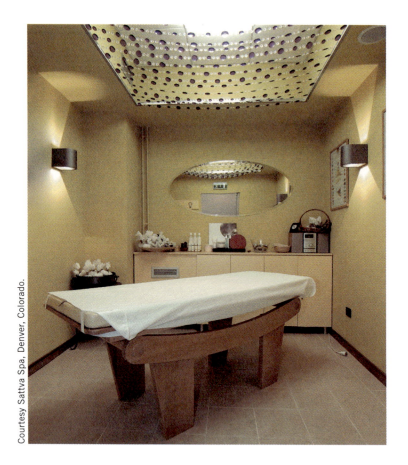

FIGURE 6-1 Treatment room should engage the senses.

Courtesy Sattva Spa, Denver, Colorado.

- Sound—What the client hears should always be pleasing and never disturbing or distracting.
- Touch—Not only the massage, but the feel of the bedding and textures that surround the client, water and product temperatures, and the air quality, including freshness, temperature, and humidity.
- Taste—A snack or beverage that may be offered to the client.
- Smell—Every aroma or odor encountered, which may be due to laundering products, the technician, or the room itself.

Effects of Stress on the Skin

Stress may exhibit itself in numerous ways on the skin. These include the following:

- Dullness (reduced cellular turnover so the skin looks dull or washed out)
- Congestion (less blood and lymphatic flow, leading to obstructions)
- Breakouts (stress triggers changes in hormonal flow, resulting in breakout)
- Sensitivities/irritation (increased cortisone secretions suppress immune system and the skin and body become more vulnerable)
- Redness (result of skin irritation above)
- Allergic reactions (from suppressed immune system)

Stress Triggers

Stress can be triggered by many things, be they internal or external. The more we are aware of them, the better we may be equipped to suggest support for a client. We can support our clients in some areas, but it is equally important to know when to refer them to a professional who can better meet their needs. These situations include many sudden or unpredictable changes in life; a more comprehensive explanation of stress triggers can be found in Chapter 10.

Some events, such as pregnancy, changes at work, or dealing with a family situation, may fall into more than one category. The predicted result is simply that stress will be present. Various stages of life will bring differing sets of stressors affecting different age groups. Daily lifestyles and environments such as school, work, or home may be a focus of stress. Social relationships rate highly as stressors, especially the formation or separation aspects. For younger groups, the competitive nature of sports or other activities may increase stress. Family conflicts can be an issue as the youth strives for ever more independence but at the same time seeks financial support. Stress for teens frequently shows up in increased skin breakouts. Estheticians can only deal with the skin symptoms and support the client by having information available for managing nutrition, wellness, and stress.

Treatment Considerations

Many facial treatments can be very effective at alleviating stress, especially those that include massage movements, but there are some things we need to keep in mind. When dealing with a client who is already experiencing high stress levels, consider selecting a treatment that focuses more on massage techniques than on aggressive exfoliation or extraction. Some of these clients may be more sensitive to sounds such as the tones associated with ultrasonic or high-frequency treatments. Others may be more sensitive to the current of galvanic or the abrasive nature of microdermabrasion. The effects of stress may cause the client to become more reactive to acid exfoliation or the temperature of towels or stones. Stress may manifest in skin with changes such as increased oil production or areas that are drier than usual. A cleansing treatment designed to rebalance the skin may be appropriate.

> **HERE'S A TIP**
>
> For some clients, use of Reiki, Ayurvedic marma-point massage, or a shirodhara treatment will bring a feeling of relaxation. Other clients may experience the shirodhara treatment as a distraction or irritation. Ensure that your legal scope of practice allows these specialized treatment types.

Skin Conditions

Skin conditions that clients present may be stable or may experience sudden or gradual changes. An acne client's skin condition may be brought gradually under control so that different treatments become advised. Inspecting the client's skin under a magnifying lamp is the best method for evaluating skin conditions and determining a treatment plan. A few simplified guidelines for treatments of specific concerns include the following:

- Redness or irritation—Select a calming, soothing treatment.
- Buildup of dead, flaky skin—Exfoliating treatment.
- Clogged pores but no redness—Exfoliate and extract.
- Broken skin, rashes, lesions—Stop treatment and reschedule or refer to a physician.
- Signs of aging—This needs a full treatment series and client goals and expectations need to be discussed.

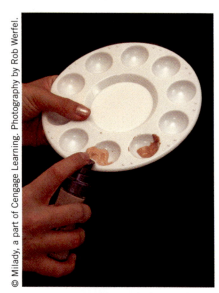

FIGURE 6–2A Dispersal of cosmetics onto a palette allows color customization.

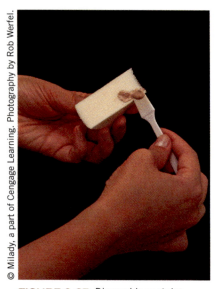

FIGURE 6–2B Disposable spatulas are an excellent tool to avoid cross contamination.

HERE'S A TIP

Some technicians prefer using fingers to brushes. In this situation, wearing gloves will prevent cross-contamination, keeps technician skin oils off the client, and still allows the warmth of the technician's hand to assist in blending applications.

Hair Removal Implications

When doing another type of treatment for the client such as hair removal, the area to be treated must be inspected for indications that could affect the treatment outcome. If the client is using an anti-aging product that makes waxing contraindicated, we must consider a safe alternative such as tweezing or sugaring, or cancelling the treatment to reschedule after the client has discontinued use of the product.

The client's tanning practices could affect the hair removal process. Ensure that the skin is completely healed after sun exposure. The client's lifestyle concerning recent and near-future sun exposure should be discussed; this includes telling the client to avoid UV radiation following the treatment, as an unexpected burn could result.

Makeup Application Implications

Makeup applications require an inspection for conditions of the skin that can impact treatment. If the client has acne, the technician may need to be more cautious about product types and focus on concealing. The client may be someone with a tattoo who would like it covered for a special occasion or photograph. If the client has freckles, the esthetician will need to discuss with the client how much coverage is desired. Signs of aging indicate the need for a careful application to avoid making lines, wrinkles, and loss of elasticity more apparent.

It is crucial that makeup artists transfer products onto a palette or disposable tray to prevent cross-contamination of the makeup products (Figure 6–2a). Viruses, cold sores, and many other forms of illness can be shared from client to client. Eye infections can occur and rapidly cause damage to an eye. No applicator should go from the client's skin back into direct contact with any product, as preventing cross-contamination is crucial to preventing contamination of products (Figure 6–2b). Sponges should be given to the client or thrown away. Cosmetic brushes should be thoroughly disinfected between clients. Mascara wands should be disposable and only dipped once into the container; never double-dip.

Lipstick should be scraped or cut off the tube and applied with a tool that can be disinfected or disposed of. Pencils must always be sharpened with a metal sharpener between clients and the metal sharpener must be disinfected. Be certain that a container is easily accessible for disposing of contaminated applicators to maintain a clean workspace at all times.

HEALTH CONDITIONS TO CONSIDER

A number of health conditions must be evaluated to determine how they will affect a treatment. Recent cosmetic intervention, including surgical or non-surgical, laser, or intense pulsed light (IPL) treatments; vision correction; pregnancy; diabetes; seizures or epilepsy; and others must all be evaluated for how they may impact the esthetic treatment. Top priority is always client safety and prevention of problems.

Recent Cosmetic Intervention

If the client has had a recent cosmetic surgical procedure, the technician must determine whether it is an indication, caution, or contraindication. Request verification from the physician that the client is approved for facial treatments. For cosmetic surgical procedures that have been performed on the area to be treated, you must always require the physician's approval or that the client have been released from physician care. Some procedures heal very quickly and treatments may be resumed in six or eight weeks; rhinoplasty and other cosmetic interventions may take a year to heal. The nose can stay very tender following rhinoplasty and it is somewhat less stable than it will be when it is healed completely.

Injectable skin and wrinkle fillers as well as Botox® can affect treatment choices. Esthetic treatments should either be done prior to the injections or be postponed a minimum of two weeks after. Gentle massage of an area that has received an injectable such as Restylane® may be beneficial for softening; however, a treatment in the area of injection could cause bruising or slow healing. If in doubt, check with the physician of the client with regard to the suitability of the treatment you wish to perform.

Laser and IPL

Intensed pulsed light (IPL) and laser treatments are commonly offered by estheticians as hair removal services. These procedures have a wide range in their impact on the skin and what treatments may be appropriate to offer the client. Some treatments may leave slightly injured skin, whereas others will have no visible effect. In general, consider skin that has been treated with IPL to be more fragile and sensitive. Wait the recommended period of time for that specific light therapy device to offer any form of facial service. No abrasive, stimulating, waxing, or exfoliating treatments should be performed without consent from a medical professional. Always be properly trained prior to using this type of device and consistently adhere to manufacturer guidelines (Figure 6–3).

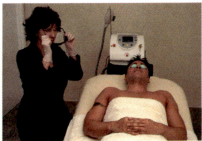

FIGURE 6–3 Follow all safety guidelines when performing IPL hair removal treatments.

© Milady, a part of Cengage Learning. Photography by Rob Werfel.

Vision Correction

Procedures to correct vision are very common today, including Lasik, cataract surgery, and multifocal lens replacement. These are very quick procedures with no visible side effects beyond dilated eyes. However, these clients may have eye sensitivities that can disappear in a few days or weeks, or linger for months. Determine whether the client has had recent eye surgery and if he or she is healing or experiencing any concerns. For those with eye sensitivities, modify treatments by avoiding product use in the eye area and taking extra care to prevent anything from getting in the eyes. Treatments such as lash perming or tinting should be postponed until the eye has returned to normal and the physician has approved the treatment or released the client.

Pregnancy

Some technicians choose never to perform treatments on pregnant clients; others may with approval of the physician. However, the condition of pregnancy will have a definite impact on services offered. Non-electrical facials might be offered, but nothing where a current flows through the body should be used. Exfoliation should be limited to products that are removed, not metabolized through the body such as BHAs. The key is to follow the guidelines of the physician for each individual. A growing trend is the medi-spa facility that focuses on treatment for pregnant clients. Within this type of facility, the presence of an on-site physician allows for client safety and appropriate treatment selection. One risk is the unfortunate chance that a client could miscarry shortly after receiving an esthetic treatment. An upset client might place responsibility on the esthetician and the service provided. The safest avenue for avoiding this type of problem is to never perform services on pregnant clients without physician approval.

Diabetes

Diabetes is a disease of the endocrine system that primarily affects the metabolism of glucose in the body. Common issues associated with all forms of diabetes are cardiovascular concerns, renal failure, and retinal damage. The changes in blood circulation may lead to slow healing and loss of sensation or pain. This is particularly common in the extremities, particularly the lower legs and feet. Clients can easily be injured in a treatment if they have low sensation and too hot a towel, stone, product, or bootie is applied. A client with diabetes may also easily develop dangerous infections any time the skin barrier is compromised.

It is important to know whether the diabetes is under control and how it is being controlled. In general, diabetics who are controlling their disease with diet will have more control and a better-performing immune system. Diabetics who must use insulin are at much higher risk. Even when the most minimal concern exists, the technician should get approval from the client's physician prior to performing treatments.

Implants

Many types of implants are surgically used in injury treatments and health issues. If the client has any dental implants, metal pins, plates, stents, pacemakers, or heart irregularities, all electrical equipment must be avoided. This particularly includes galvanic, high-frequency, ultrasonic, or any other device where current flows through the body. Non-electrical treatments may be offered and approval of a physician should be sought if any concerns are present.

Seizures or Epilepsy

In the event a client suffers from neurological disorders such as epilepsy or unexplained seizures, avoid all electrical treatments and all light-related treatments. These clients may have an episode triggered either by electrical current or by lights. Although only 1 in 20 people who have epilepsy has seizures triggered by flashing lights, avoiding the use of light therapies on this group of clients is a safety consideration.

Allergies

Clients who suffer from allergies need a thorough consultation. An esthetician must find out what types of allergies they have; some may be food-related,

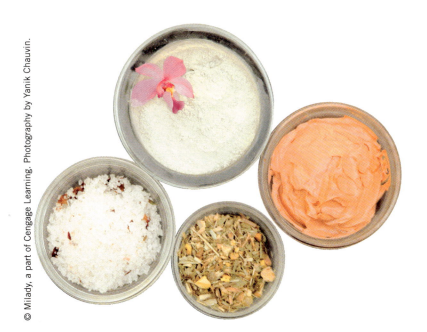

© Milady, a part of Cengage Learning. Photography by Yanik Chauvin.

FIGURE 6–4 Always investigate ingredients to avoid allergic reactions as many products contain natural ingredients.

topical, or airborne. Some people who cannot eat a substance cannot have it applied topically, either. Citrus fruits are an excellent example of this. If a client gets hives from eating citrus fruits, then the technician would want to avoid all products with any form of citrus as an ingredient. This can require some homework, as ingredients and their derivatives are not always clearly explained (Figure 6–4). If we apply linden, a common and calming botanical, to a client who is allergic to citrus, the client may have an allergic reaction, as linden is obtained from the numerous Tilia, or lime tree, species.

A person who suffers from hay fever allergies may be more reactive to products when symptoms are more prevalent. Avoid known allergenic substances and treat the client as having sensitive skin. Many times, the medications taken for allergies will cause the skin to be more dehydrated; the skin will benefit from hydrating and soothing treatments.

Of growing concern are allergies to latex substances. Reactions may range from immediate reaction to delayed hypersensitivity. Some reactions can be mild, with the presence of itching and redness of the skin; others may result in anaphylactic shock. It is important that an esthetician be aware of all sources of latex, including gloves, bandages, and some sponges. When a latex allergy is present, food allergies are also often present to items such as banana, kiwi, papaya, avocado, and apricot.

Autoimmune Disorders

An autoimmune disorder is a condition that occurs when the immune system mistakenly attacks and destroys healthy body tissue. There are many different forms, including multiple sclerosis, rheumatoid arthritis, and lupus. If any autoimmune disorder is present, avoid all stimulating or harsh treatments. These disorders are generally progressive, so we must be prepared to stay abreast of the physician's advice and adapt treatments to meet the client's changing needs.

MEDICATIONS THAT MAY AFFECT TREATMENT CHOICE

Many times, visible changes in the skin may be a direct result of medications the client is taking. Every time we see a client, we must update our knowledge of any medications they may be taking and any changes in dosage. A technician who is informed about the medications a client is taking and what the possible side effects of those medications may be is in a better position to assist the client. Be sure you review with the client all sources of medications, as listed below.

- Over-the-counter medications
- Prescription medications
- Vitamins
- Homeopathic remedies
- Patches, or implanted medications
- Topical medications

If the client has started on a new drug that you are not familiar with, an excellent source to consult is a printed drug reference guide or an Internet site such as www.webmd.com. These should provide you with a complete listing of skin concerns or side effects. Provided here is a listing of common oral prescription drugs (Table 6–1):

CATEGORY OF DRUG	COMMON DRUG NAMES	COMMON REASONS FOR PRESCRIPTION
Antidepressants	Prozac®, Zoloft®	Depression
Antivirals	Zovirax®, Valtrex®	Prevent or treat herpes simplex (cold sores)
Antibiotics	Tetracycline	Acne or infections
Antifungals	Lamisil®	Fungal infections
Diuretics	Hydrochlorothiazide	Hypertension
Hormones	Estrogen	Menopause symptoms
Hypoglycemic agents	Actos®, Glucophage®	Diabetes
Birth control medications	Many varieties	Prevent pregnancy

TABLE 6–1 Common Oral Prescription Drugs.

Provided here is a listing of common topical prescription drugs (Table 6–2):

CATEGORY OF DRUG	COMMON DRUG NAMES	COMMON REASONS FOR PRESCRIPTION
Anti-aging drugs	Renova®	Lines and wrinkles
Antibiotics	Cleocin T®	Acne
Antivirals	Denavir®, Zovax®	Cold sores
Anti-inflammatory drugs	Aclovate®	Irritation from peel or treatment

TABLE 6–2 Common Topical Prescription Drugs.

© Milady, a part of Cengage Learning

There are many different types of drugs and they fall into many different categories depending on the condition they are designed to treat. Every year, new drugs are brought to market to add to the choices the physician may recommend or to perform better or with fewer side effects. What is not commonly realized is how many skin effects can be a result of these medications. See Appendix A for a more complete set of tables that show common drugs and their skin effects. Concerning treatment selection, if a client is not exhibiting any skin issues from a drug, treatments may be performed. The client should be monitored and caution exercised if any skin changes are noted, with a few specific exemptions.

If the client is using Accutane®, Retin-A®, Renova™, Tazorac®, Differin®, or another skin-thinning or exfoliating drug, specific treatment criteria must be followed. Thinner skin can last as long as a full year following discontinuation of Accutane. For the other drugs listed, a client should have completed the prescription cycle and no longer be taking the medications several weeks before the following treatments are performed:

- All waxing
- Exfoliating treatments
- Peels
- Stimulating treatments

For numerous classes of medication, side effects may include skin itching, bruising, rashes, hives, peeling, or photosensitivity. There is a risk that these could manifest during or after a treatment in which the skin is exposed to a number of products. Determining the history of possible reactions associated with a treatment and then educating the client as to possible side effects can impact what treatment will be selected. The types of drugs that these reactions are seen with include the following:

- Anti-anxiety drugs
- Anticonvulsants
- Antidepressants
- Antipsychotics
- General nervous system stimulants
- Sedatives
- Beta blockers
- Calcium channel blockers
- Nitrates
- Anti-arrhythmics
- Antihypertensives
- Antihistamines
- Anti-asthmatics
- Bronchodilators
- Lipid-lowering drugs
- Antiplatelets
- Hormones
- Birth control medications
- Antiulcer drugs

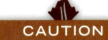

CAUTION

Clients who are taking oral steroids like prednisone should avoid all treatments that are stimulating or exfoliating; this includes any form of waxing.

CAUTION

Clients taking blood thinners should avoid extraction or waxing. Common blood thinners include Coumadin (warfarin) and heparin.

Any time a client comes in who has recently started taking a new medication, the skin response must be closely monitored. Always document this monitoring to use for future comparisons.

LIFESTYLE EFFECTS ON TREATMENT CHOICE

An esthetician should practice quality training and use cautious judgment when performing treatments. However, we have little control over a client's lifestyle. Daily practices and activities both before and after the treatment have a strong impact on the potential outcome.

Case Study

A male client comes into the clinic requesting a hair removal treatment on his back. He is a regular client and routinely has the hair removed from his arms and shoulders and the random patches that grow on his back by use of wax. This client prefers to maintain a tan, and in preparation for his vacation he has recently been visiting a tanning booth. The esthetician has informed and cautioned the client about possible risks involved. The client explains he last used the tanning booth two days prior. The service is performed as requested, but the client is cautioned again about the avoidance of tanning for several days.

The client returns the following week, unhappy with the treatment due to the hyperpigmented brown patches on his back. The client had felt the esthetician's cautions were not that important and visited the tanning facility the day following the hair removal service. The hair removal had resulted in exfoliated areas of skin, increasing the likelihood of sunburn and development of dark patches. This was worsened by his sun exposure while on vacation. He also admitted to having used the tanning booth prior to coming in for waxing. This is a common example of how a client's lifestyle may affect the outcome of a treatment.

Outdoor Lifestyles

Lifestyle activities affect the treatments that are appropriate for each client. It is critical that we find out about clients' recent activities and future plans. Estheticians need to know the clients' hobbies and how their free time is spent. Those who love to spend time outdoors are not good candidates for exfoliating or other stimulating treatments. Hair removal services must be performed on them with great caution. Clients may sometimes withhold information in their desire to have a specific service. Clients might not feel it is important to discuss plans to go backpacking, hiking, or horseback riding in their desire to have a peel done. Clients may not realize that it is just as risky to be outdoors watching a game of golf as it is to be golfing. For this reason, the informed consent and agreement to application is a crucial document. It should include a statement that clients sign. agreeing to follow all pre- and post-treatment guidelines, which are to be clearly spelled out. Selecting the right services for clients and their lifestyles is a joint effort that must have support from both technicians and clients.

Smokers

Clients who smoke present special issues to the esthetician. They may have skin goals that are not achievable due to their lifestyle choice. A treatment may make their skin feel better temporarily, but as long as they are smoking, damage to the skin will continue to occur. The esthetician must clearly explain this to the client and set achievable goals. A client's feeling that he or she is paying for unsuccessful treatments may result in a negative financial impact for the esthetician. It is better to be honest with these clients and stick to realistic goals.

Special Occasions

If a client has a special occasion coming up, treatment services must be carefully planned to limit risks of a negative reaction (Figure 6–5). The client may desire to receive a treatment at the last minute in order to look his or her best, when in fact this may be a poor choice. Hair removal should be done in advance so that any rash or irritation can be dealt with. Exfoliating treatments should be completed in advance and should never be combined with waxing services in the same area. Plan accordingly and stagger the services to get the best result and the fewest possible reactions.

Brides or those attending a special occasion will sometimes want hair removal and makeup on the day of the wedding. To minimize the risk of complications, complete all hair removal treatments a minimum of 48 hours in advance. Any redness or irritation will have had the opportunity to subside and the makeup will apply more smoothly.

Make sure that the client has the proper products to deal with any issues that might arise from the treatments offered. Exfoliation and waxing clients should receive some sort of post-peel product to deal with redness or irritation.

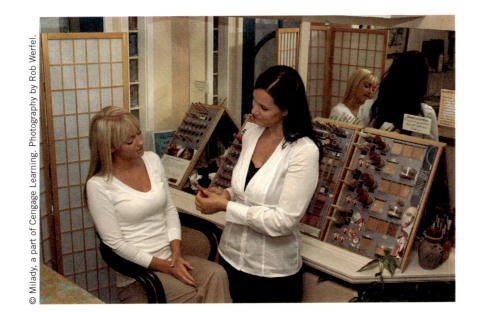

© Milady, a part of Cengage Learning. Photography by Rob Werfel.

FIGURE 6–5 Special occasions require advance planning of treatments and applications.

Clients have the best skin results for class reunions, social gatherings, and other special occasions when treatments start in advance in order to get the skin into optimum condition. This should always be used in conjunction with the appropriate home care. Client consulting and education will help achieve this. A specific skin goal will guide the esthetician to the appropriate treatment choice.

Physical Limitations

Recent injuries are always a consideration. If the client has had a shoulder, hip, or back injury, consider whether they will be able to change garments, to get on and off the treatment lounge, and to be comfortable for the duration of the treatment.

When providing body treatments, this is equally critical. In some treatments, it is necessary for the client to turn over or to get up and use the shower. Pain from injury or health conditions could impact this. Communicate about what the client can easily accomplish and alter treatment accordingly. Shoulder injuries are common in older clients; this may impair clients' ability to change clothes but not their desire for a treatment. The solution is to provide them with something easy to put on: no snaps, ties, buttons, or Velcro, or to protect their street clothing and limit treatments strictly to the face. For some technicians, this will mean changing their massage, but even the more limited facial may benefit the client's skin and mental attitude. An adjustable bed or bolsters can also help with client comfort. Modifying treatments to meet client needs can help keep clients younger longer by supporting a positive mental outlook. Make efforts to always accommodate the special needs of a client.

CONTRAINDICATIONS

In some situations we cannot offer treatment to a client, and in others specific treatments are contraindicated. It is critical that we know when not to perform requested treatments, as the health and safety of the client must always be of primary concern. One positive development is that modern medical treatments and advances have lifted some contraindications. For example, mitral valve prolapse (MVP) was in the past a contraindication for some treatments, as clients with the condition are more prone to infections. Now the medical guidelines have changed and these clients no longer are considered to be contraindicated or to require pre-medication for certain services such as permanent cosmetics. If in doubt about the safety of any treatment for a client, it is always important to request that the client get clearance from a physician in writing prior to performing the service.

Occasionally, a client will come in for a treatment and the consultation reveals contraindications. A contraindication is an indication that, due to specific concerns, a treatment would not be advisable and may deliver unpredictable results. If the client presents with a skin condition that is not a routine, esthetically treatable one, it is important to ask if the client has seen a doctor for it. If so, the technician needs to know the diagnosis to determine if it is safe to proceed with the treatment. If the client has not seen a physician, the treatment should be postponed until after an examination by a medical practitioner.

Any visible skin irritation or rash should be considered a contraindication. Community-acquired Methicillin-resistant *Staphylococcus aureus* (MRSA) is highly contagious bacterial skin infection typified by a sudden occurrence of small red bumps. This progresses to inflamed and swollen, red and painful skin. Clients with any contagious disease should be rescheduled to protect the technician, staff, and other clients. A client with a cough could have a chronic condition, be recovering from a cold or other virus that could be shared, or suffer from some other dormant medical condition. It is appropriate to ask and get the necessary information to offer or decline a service. Other specific contagious diseases could include active herpes, ringworm, or oozing poison oak, sumac, or ivy.

Manufacturer Guidelines

Some manufacturers explicitly call out certain medical conditions as contraindicated for specific treatments or protocols. These manufacturer guidelines should always be strictly adhered to and never altered. If in doubt as to why a manufacturer would list a condition as contraindicated, contact the manufacturer for more information. As noted above, certain medications and health conditions can interact with treatments, causing increased risk for the client.

State Guidelines

Some states specifically prohibit estheticians from working with certain medical conditions. These conditions are commonly the presence of rashes, skin conditions, or illness. Adherence to state guidelines is always required for contraindications, even if they may seem excessive.

Eye Issues

Conjunctivitis, sometimes called pinkeye due to the redness of the eye, can be caused by viruses, bacteria, chemical fumes, irritation or allergies, and possibly excessive tearing. As there is no way for an esthetician to determine the cause of the conjunctivitis, any treatment should be rescheduled. The viral and bacterial forms are highly contagious.

A person with a viral form of conjunctivitis should stay home until symptoms clear. In general, no medication is used to treat viruses. A person with a bacterial form can return to work 24 hours following the start of an antibiotic. However, any treatment would still be contraindicated until the eye has returned to normal to ensure client comfort and to avoid aggravating the condition.

HIV and Hepatitis

The bloodborne pathogen HIV, human immunodeficiency virus, can eventually lead to the development of AIDS, or acquired immune deficiency syndrome. This may take many years to develop, and although treatments are improving, there is not yet a cure. Symptoms can vary but often include weakness, fever, sore throat, nausea, headaches, diarrhea, a white coating on the tongue, weight loss, and swollen lymph nodes.

In the past, estheticians have been concerned about contracting HIV from a client; however, updated information shows that this risk is very low if the client is otherwise in good health and not experiencing issues such as rashes, visible sores, or other wounds. Clients with open sores, cuts, abrasions, acne, or any form of damaged or broken skin such as sunburn or blisters could pass the virus to another person through direct contact. Bloodborne pathogens may also be transmitted through the mucous membranes of the eyes, nose, and mouth. If the client is not experiencing any skin conditions, the more pressing concern is whether the treatment puts the client at risk. When the immune system is compromised, no treatment that could create a wound should be performed. This would include peels, microdermabrasion, and waxing, unless specifically approved by a physician.

It is much easier to contract some forms of hepatitis, an inflammation of the liver, than it is to contract HIV. The symptoms of acute hepatitis are flulike and may manifest as quickly as two weeks or as long as six to nine months after infection. This is a problem for the Centers for Disease Control (CDC), as the source of the infection is usually difficult to trace. It is best to always reschedule any client who is not feeling well, as the possibility of spreading contagious illness exists.

Non-Contagious Contraindications

Most contraindications occur to due a client's being contagious, but some non-contagious indicators mean that treatment is not recommended in some situations. Always be cautious when working with an electrical current that travels into the skin and avoid use on clients with braces, metal implants, or a pacemaker. Also avoid these types of procedures on any client with epilepsy, pregnancy, high blood pressure, fevers, or any infections. Effects of diabetes may have progressed to lower nerve sensitivity, so electrical current should also be avoided with diabetic patients. Clients who suffer from migraines or epilepsy should avoid highly stimulating treatments to prevent triggering an episode.

In the treatment room, we may encounter clients with both indications and contraindications for treatment. In this situation, the contraindications must supersede the client's requests for the service. A foremost consideration must always be to do no harm to the client, and if a treatment is questionable or not advised, do not perform it.

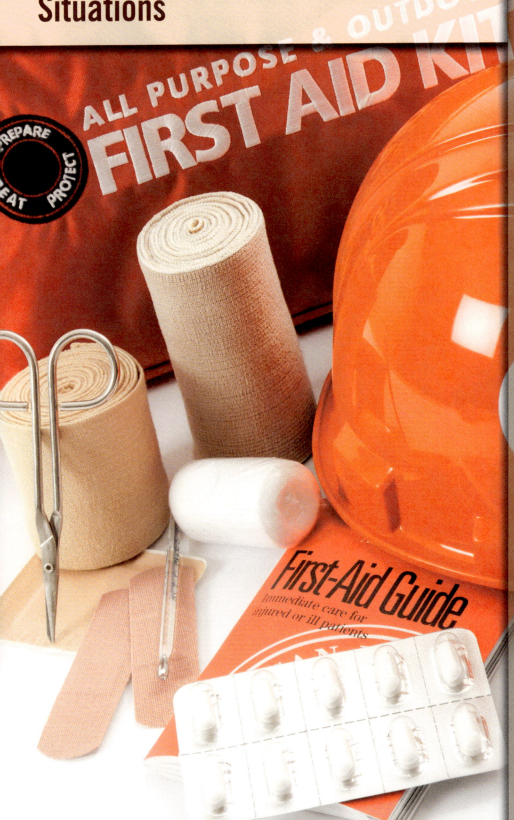

CHAPTER

7

Emergency & Non-Emergency Situations

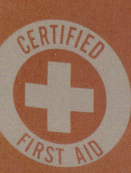

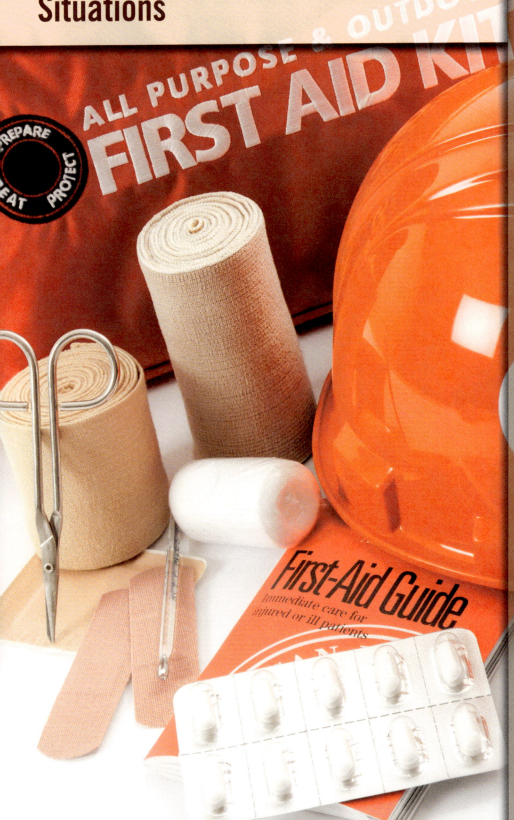

INTRODUCTION

An emergency will often occur without any forewarning or expectations. Emergency situations can range from natural disasters and weather conditions to medical concerns. Non-emergency situations may involve unexpected weather conditions that are not severe but should be closely monitored (Figure 7–1). Dealing with emergency and non-emergency situations successfully in the clinic depends on preparedness. It is imperative to be prepared by developing protocols and pursuing continuing education. In an urgent situation, being properly equipped mentally and structurally will allow the thought process to flow without panic.

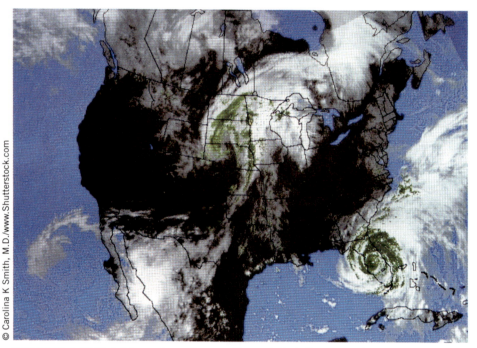

© Carolina K Smith, M.D./www.Shutterstock.com

FIGURE 7–1 Monitor daily weather patterns and forecasts for better preparedness.

Business owners should take the time to develop the necessary emergency action plans specifically for their structure and business operations. Require that all employees be trained in how to respond when faced with a crisis. Emergency and non-emergency situations may result in the loss of utilities on which your business depends for continued daily operations. Within your emergency action plan, prepare alternate methods to consider in the event that power or water supplies are lost. Having knowledge and plans for alternate methods will prevent clients in mid-treatment from being put at risk. Also consider developing manual procedures in case electrical power is lost and your business uses computer software or an electricity-dependent system for financial transactions.

DISASTER SITUATIONS

A natural disaster that may be predictable to some extent may include a hurricane or tornado (Figures 7–2a, 7–2b, 7–2c, and 7–2d). This type of weather condition is commonly preceded by storm watches or warnings. A watch may occur when conditions indicate a storm is likely, and a warning indicates that a storm has developed. Other forms of natural disasters generally occur without any expectation; earthquakes and landslides are perfect examples of this.

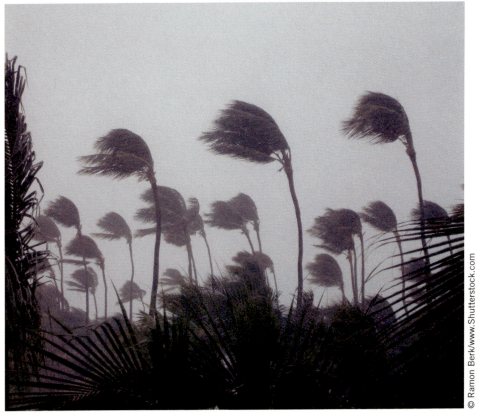

FIGURE 7–2A Hurricane.

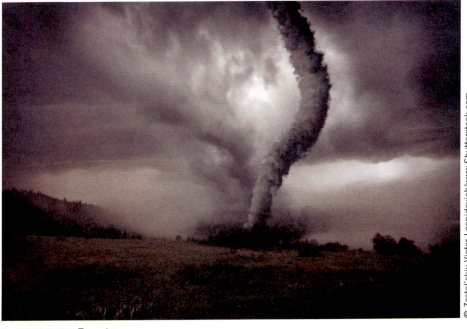

FIGURE 7–2B Tornado.

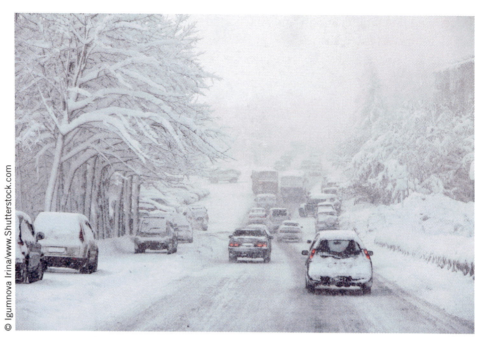

© Igumnova Irina/www.Shutterstock.com

FIGURE 7–2C Snowstorm.

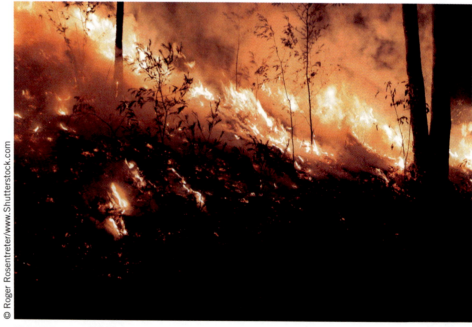

© Roger Rosentreter/www.Shutterstock.com

FIGURE 7–2D Wildfire.

Be familiar with your local area and understand which types of natural disasters are most likely. Being aware of local weather patterns and seasonal changes will allow you to be prepared in most any situation.

Disaster Planning

Numerous resources are available for determining local weather patterns (average temperatures, rainfall, and types of common storms) or if any geographical or climate hazards exist (earthquakes, wildfires, or flooding). Some notable resources include the following:

- National Oceanic and Atmospheric Administration (NOAA): www.noaa.gov
- NOAA National Weather Service: www.weather.gov
- NOAA Storm Prediction Center: www.spc.noaa.gov
- U.S. Geological Survey (emergencies and disasters): www.usgs.gov

In addition, some resources that provide information on preparedness for a natural disaster include:

- Ready.gov: www.ready.gov
- American Red Cross (preparedness link) www.redcross.org
- Federal Emergency Management Agency (FEMA): www.fema.gov

Being properly equipped for potential natural disasters is a vital element of offering a safe environment for clients and fellow employees. Keeping a stocked emergency preparedness kit will assist you when dealing with an unexpected situation. This emergency supply kit should be stored in a clearly labeled, airtight container and placed in an easily accessed location. The Federal Emergency Management Agency (FEMA) provides a list of recommended supplies, which you may need to adjust for local geographical or weather events (Figure 7–3).

Flashlight and Extra Batteries

- Portable battery-powered or hand-cranked radio
- A listing of essential resources and contacts:
    - Local radio stations and frequencies _____
    - Local emergency broadcast television _____
    - Non-emergency police support number _____
    - Gas leak hotline _____

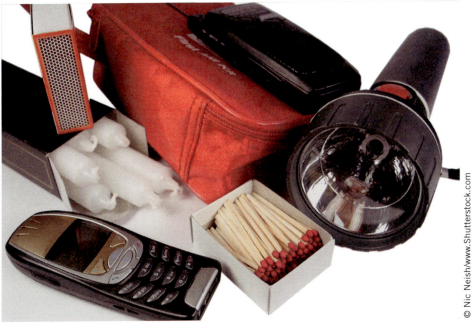

© Nic Neish/www.Shutterstock.com

FIGURE 7–3 Emergency supplies.

- Locksmith _____
- County sheriff _____
- State patrol _____
- Transportation assistance _____
- Emergency contacts of employees _____
- Whistle (for signaling for help)
- Well-stocked first-aid kit and manual
- Face masks (to filter dust and pathogens)
- Blankets
- Nonperishable food items
- Water (approximately one gallon per person per day)
- Nonelectric can opener
- Essential medications
- Small toolkit (may be needed to turn off utilities)
- Hand sanitizer or moist towelettes
- Garbage bags
- Sturdy shoes

You may find it beneficial to keep other items such as a change of clothing, toothbrush and toiletries in your car or office. You may become stranded, and these items can be beneficial to safety and personal comfort.

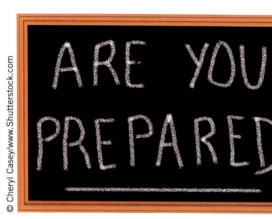

© Cheryl Casey/www.Shutterstock.com

FIGURE 7–4 Are you prepared?

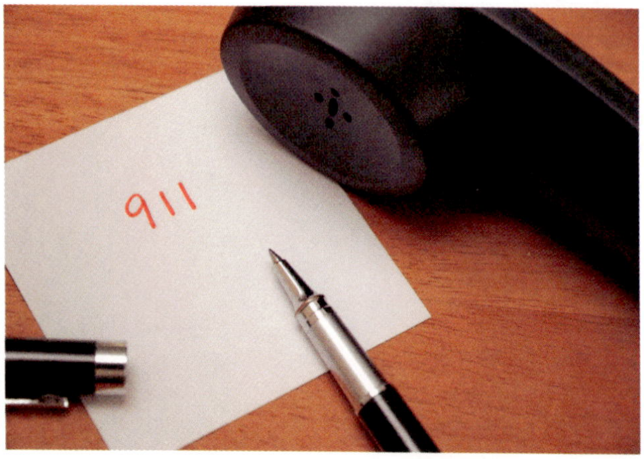

© Gnohz/www.Shutterstock.com

FIGURE 7–5 Call 9-1-1 for emergency assistance.

In the event that you are confronted with a natural disaster situation, the following points will be helpful (Figure 7–4):

- Stay calm (use deep breathing if necessary).
- Watch the television, listen to the radio, or check the Internet for current alerts.
- Be aware of nearby storm conditions.
- Move to a safe location such as an interior room (severe storms), or under a sturdy doorframe or beneath furniture (earthquake).
- Stay away from windows or other glass items such as shelving.
- If a treatment is being performed and conditions warrant stopping the service, promptly remove any products from the skin and assist your client to a safe location of the clinic. (Allow the client to put on a robe if necessary.)
- In a flood situation, do not drink tap water until local authorities have issued approval.
- Do not attempt to drive through a flooded area.
- Beware of any dropped electrical lines.
- Do not attempt to use an elevator.

9-1-1

Generally, if there is a situation that may be perceived as a medical or violent emergency, call 9-1-1 or your local number for emergency services (Figure 7–5).

9-1-1 service is a vital part of our nation's emergency response and disaster preparedness system. If you have trouble getting through on a cell phone, try a landline. The Federal Communications Commission (FCC) has the following recommendations when calling 9-1-1 for assistance:

- Tell the emergency operator the exact location of the emergency.
- Describe the nature of the emergency.
- Give the emergency operator the number you are calling from so that if you get disconnected they can call you back.
- Many areas offer enhanced or E9-1-1 services, which means the dispatch office you are connected to can retrieve your number and location. If your locality does not offer E9-1-1, make sure you know the location and the number you are calling from.

Building Structure

Your individual facility is of primary concern in establishing your safety and evacuation plan. Countless scenarios may be encountered that involve your building structure. Some of the factors that should be considered for your building and/or business include the following items:

- Location
- Type of construction
- Ground level or other
- Location of doors and types of locks on doors
- Location of windows
- Location of telephones, flashlights, fire extinguishers
- Location of AEDs, first-aid supplies, eye-wash stations
- Security system/emergency alert systems
- Wet rooms and changing areas

It is critical that for any door that locks there be a master key available in the main control area of the clinic. A protocol should be in place to protect client privacy, but also to intervene in case of emergency. An esthetician performing a treatment or a client in a restroom or dressing room could encounter a health concern or need immediate assistance. Make efforts to protect client privacy, but intervention may be necessary in a serious situation.

Evacuation

You may be faced with a building or area evacuation. You can contact your local authorities in the event that there is a widespread evacuation, but it is your responsibility to be prepared if your workplace faces evacuation. This could be in the event of a fire or structural concern. Several factors should be contemplated when developing a business evacuation plan, including the following:

- Have a system for knowing who—employees and clients both—is in the building at all times.
- Identify who is responsible for shutting down critical operations and locking the door in the event of an evacuation.

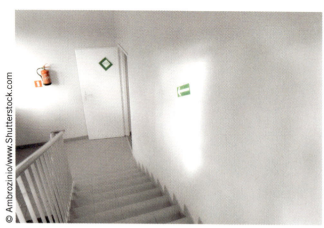

FIGURE 7–6 Know the location of emergency exit routes.

- Locate and make copies of building and site maps with critical utilities and exit routes clearly marked (Figure 7–6).
- Plan two exit routes from every point and designate a meeting site; this will allow you to verify that everyone is accounted for.

It is crucial to have a plan for both medical emergency and non-emergency situations. The incidents of September 11, 2001, serve as a harsh reminder that each of us has to be prepared to deal with the unexpected. Disasters are non-discriminatory. Those who respond with a calm mind and a clear plan help themselves and others survive.

Transportation

In the event that you are performing a service or treatment off-site, some factors of special consideration may need to be examined in questionable weather. These same issues may also be relevant to consider when giving a client directions to your facility.

- Ensure that directions to your facility or the work locations are clear, concise, and easy to understand.
- Have backup transportation available; public services or a willing friend will suffice.
- Perform routine maintenance on your vehicle, including checking the air pressure of the tires and oil levels.
- Have a charged cell phone in the event of an emergency.
- Always be aware of weather and road conditions.

Driving a client is high liability; try to avoid this if your assistance is requested. If the client needs to seek medical care, call 9-1-1 or a family member.

NON-DISASTER PROTOCOLS

A protocol is a plan or written guide with steps organized in simplified and sequential order for a specific situation. These could be listed in a handbook provided to each new team member or as a separate section in your written safety plan. To be readily available at any given time, consider having a copy of this both at the front desk and in the dispensary. It is recommended that you have both your lawyer and your insurance provider review and consult with you on the finished protocols.

Some specific protocols that would be useful for an esthetic clinic but not discussed elsewhere in this book include issues of criminal activity. This may include dealing with an intruder, theft, or violence. It could be a frightening experience to be unexpectedly faced with an intruder. Having proper training and knowing the protocols will allow you to think more clearly and know what to do in unanticipated situations.

HERE'S A TIP

Develop an emergency action plan that includes emergency escape routes and evacuation procedures. Regularly practice timed drills to ensure that all employees know the most efficient routes for evacuating the area in the event of a fire, hazardous materials, environmental threats, or building system failures. Train staff in the emergency action plan and post diagrams showing the escape routes for clients.

Intruders

Though it is uncommon, a clinic may experience an intruder at some point. An intruder can be described as any unwelcome person; intruders may or may not have criminal intentions. It is worth your time to have a simple plan for dealing with an intruder. An intruder may enter your clinic during normal business operations or during hours when no one is present. The intruder may be there for purposes of theft or vandalism, or because of personal relationship issues.

Burglary

An intruder who has a purpose of theft or robbery may appear during regular operational hours or when the business is closed. Your personal safety, as well as that of your clients, can be quickly compromised. Taking prevention measures and knowing how best to conduct your actions in the event a burglary occurs can be helpful in averting a bad situation. Some generalized points are listed here, but developing relationships with your local police department will assist you in developing a more specific and individualized plan.

- Have at least two employees open and close the business.
- Do not release personal information to strangers.
- Keep purses and personal valuables locked in desks or lockers.
- Install a robbery alarm.
- Vary times and routes of travel for bank deposits.
- Don't use marked "money bags" that make it obvious to would-be robbers that you are carrying money for deposit.
- Keep a low balance in the cash register.
- Place excess money in a safe or deposit it at your bank as soon as possible.
- Cooperate with the robber for your own safety and the safety of others. Comply with a robber's demands. Remain calm and think clearly. Make mental notes of the robber's physical description and other observations important to law enforcement officers.
- If you have a silent alarm and can reach it without being noticed, use it. Otherwise, wait until the robber leaves.
- Be careful. Most robbers are just as nervous as you are.
- Stay alert! Know who is in your business and where they are. Be aware of suspicious activity outside your place of business. Write down license numbers of suspicious vehicles if visible from inside your business.
- Make sure the sales counter can be seen clearly from the outside. Don't put up advertisements, flyers, displays, signs, posters or other items on windows or doors that might obstruct the view of the register from inside or outside your business.
- Try to greet clients as they enter your business. Look them in the eye and ask them if they need help. Your attention can discourage a robber.

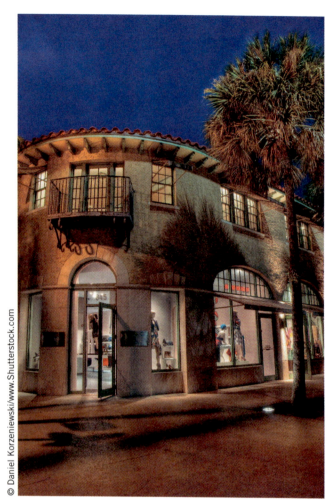

FIGURE 7-7 Keep your business well-lit after dark.

- Keep your business well lit inside and out. Employees should report any burned-out lights to the business owner or manager. Keep trees and bushes trimmed so they don't block any outdoor lights (Figure 7–7).
- Encourage the police to stop by your business.
- Use care after dark. Be cautious when exiting the clinic or taking out the trash at night. Make sure another employee inside the business keeps you within eyesight while you are involved in work details outside your building.
- If you see something suspicious, call the police. Never try to handle it yourself. It could cost you your life.
- Handle cash carefully. Avoid making your business a tempting target for robbers. Move all large bills right away by placing underneath a cash drawer or into a safe. If a customer tries to pay with a large bill, politely ask if he or she has a smaller one. Explain that you keep very little cash on hand.
- Leave blinds and drapes partially open during closing hours.
- Make sure that important signs stay posted. For example, the front door should bear signs that say, "Employees Cannot Open the Time-Lock Safe."
- If your business is robbed, put your safety first. Your personal safety is more important than money or merchandise.

If a robbery occurs, contact 9-1-1 once the person has left and provide them with all the details. Be prepared to answer extensive and specific questions. Consulting with local enforcement officials will help determine the best safety protocols for your possible situations. Be sure you promptly contact your insurance provider to report any loss.

The use of computerized technology can be very helpful in business operations. Unfortunately, this equipment can be quite expensive, making it desirable in a robbery. It is a good idea to invest in some form of data backup and store this separately on a secondary storage drive or off-site. Client and staff privacy are also of concern, so make sure personal history files and employment records that may contain personal or sensitive information are kept locked or in an otherwise secure situation.

Internal Theft

Another often overlooked intrusion of a business is sometimes the most difficult to deal with, and that is internal loss. Protocols must be in place to keep all staff members accountable and reduce temptation and risk by minimizing opportunity. This type of theft can be difficult to prevent and prosecute. Use caution that only highly trusted staff members have access to financial records, credit cards, cash, and checks. Watch closely for signs of inventory loss or unexplained cash shortages (Figure 7–8). One common means of internal theft may include pilfering products and supplies. Maintaining inventory control procedures will allow quick notice of any changes. Another type of internal theft may result from excess discounts being given when charging for treatments. It is important to have a policy regarding discounts and their use.

Violence

Workplace violence can be described as any act of physical violence, threats of physical violence, harassment, intimidation, or other threatening, disruptive behavior that occurs at the worksite. Workplace violence can affect or involve clients, employees, or management.

A number of different actions in the work environment can trigger workplace violence. Such violence may even be the result of non-work-related situations such as personal relationships or the emotional buildup from experiencing a bad day. Whatever the cause and whoever the perpetrator, workplace violence is not to be accepted or tolerated.

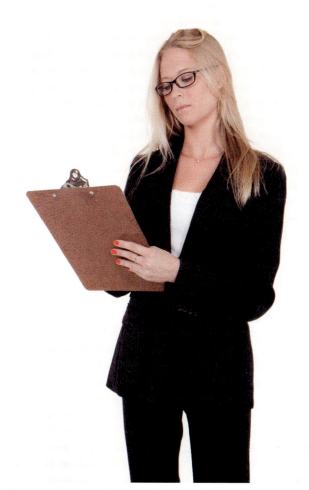

FIGURE 7–8 Conducting a regular product inventory is one method of preventing internal theft.

There is no sure way to predict human behavior, and while there may be warning signs, there is no specific profile of a potentially dangerous individual. The best prevention comes from identifying problems early and dealing with them. An excellent resource on workplace violence is published by the U.S. Department of Agriculture (USDA) will be found at the Web site www.usda.gov/news/pubs/violence/wpv.htm. This link contains a detailed handbook dealing with workplace violence prevention and response.

Stalking may occur during working hours and is defined as the crime of harassing someone with persistent, inappropriate, and unwanted attention. This can be a form of violent behavior and a cause for concern in the operation of a business. In the event that you feel that you, a coworker, or a client may be the victim of a stalker, a few key points may be important:

- Document as many specific incidents as possible, including time, date, and description of the concern.
- Contact local authorities to discuss your situation.
- Don't be too nice. You can't reason with a stalker and they may mistake your kindness for an invitation for continued contact.
- Notify coworkers, neighbors, and friends so they are aware if any unusual activity occurs.
- Never walk alone in dark or isolated areas during the day or night.

- If you have a photo of the stalker, share it with coworkers, neighbors, and friends.
- Protect your privacy—don't give out personal information unless absolutely necessary.

Everyone can be faced with emergency and non-emergency situations, which may occur in a wide variety of forms. Work on developing the necessary plans or protocols to ensure a safe workplace is offered for all employees and clients. Provide all staff members with the information and encourage their input. Take the time to practice drills and to check supplies in emergency kits at least twice a year.

Situations in the Treatment Room

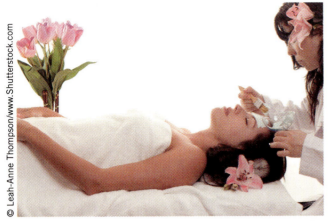

FIGURE 8-1 Proper communication is essential to prevention of problems.

INTRODUCTION

Any time a treatment is being performed on a client, unexpected situations can occur. Learning how to handle specific treatment room situations is an ongoing process as new techniques are practiced and new products and various modalities incorporated. Professional responsibility requires the professional to seek continuing education. Being informed on the progression within the industry will help you to be better prepared in any situation. It is also important to educate clients so that they are informed about what may occur (Figure 8–1).

It is a good idea for every skin care practice to have some form of an internal alert system. With this alert system, an esthetician can get assistance if needed, without leaving the client. The system could use beepers, an intercom, or even cell phones. Whatever method is used should be quick and employed without panic so that no undue stress is caused to other guests. In the case of a treatment room emergency, however, you can't afford to be too polite and put the client at risk. If no other method is available, summon assistance from other staff. Do this in a voice that will get attention but not sound frantic. All staff members should be trained to immediately assist should this or another preestablished alert signal be called out.

Three types of situations can happen in a treatment room: consequences, side effects, and complications. It is important that you be able separate these in your mind and that they be covered in client pre-treatment information and on the informed consent form.

CONSEQUENCES OF TREATMENTS

The dictionary defines a consequence as a direct result of some action or event, something that necessarily results from a particular set of conditions. In our esthetic world, skin turning pink from stimulation is a consequence. This is unavoidable and to be expected with certain treatments. Examples of stimulation that can cause skin reddening include:

- Waxing
- Massage
- Peels
- Microdermabrasion
- Steam
- Brushes
- Hot towels
- Hot stones

These are just a few examples. We trigger the skin flushing with many of our services due to an increase in circulation or because of exposure to increased temperatures. Skin turning pink to red in the treatment room is a predictable response. It tells us that the skin is responding and that we are bringing fresh blood and nourishment into the area. In the case of pinkness during a facial treatment, it is even a desired result. Some clients turn pink very easily and others hardly change color at all. This is due to the natural tone and amount of melanin in the skin.

During the consultation process, it is important to find out if a client's skin turns pink during stimulating exercise and how quickly it calms down. This can be an indicator of how the skin will respond during a treatment. Ask the client if he or she flushes or blushes easily; this will indicate how likely it is that the skin will turn red quickly due to skin stimulation (Figure 8–2). It is important to let the client know that flushed skin is a possibil-

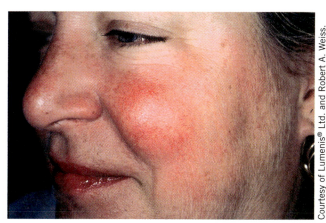

FIGURE 8–2 Some clients may tend to naturally blush with little stimulation.

ity when the treatment is completed. The client is probably used to this so it won't come as a shock, but the reminder will allow the client to be mentally prepared.

Other consequences can be a little more intimidating for both the technician and the client. Advising the client of the possible consequences of the treatment is part of performing the service.

Hair Removal

Hair removal is a common treatment offered as an esthetic service. Increasingly, both men and women are having body hair removed. Discomfort and reddening of the skin are expected consequences of this service, regardless of the method used (Figure 8–3). Other consequences exist, but these may be minimized by proper communication of client skin care pre- and post-treatment.

The client must be educated to avoid tanning before and after the service. The method of removal to be used determines how long that period must be. For waxing, 48 to 72 hours prior to and following the treatment are generally enough. If laser or IPL is to be used, there can be no tanning for at least two weeks prior to the treatment. Estheticians normally mention this restriction to clients but may not offer a thorough explanation. It is important to point out that not following the guidelines could lead to increased sensitivity, burns, and the risk of hyperpigmentation.

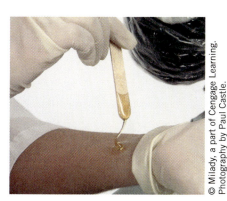

FIGURE 8–3 Test the temperature of heated wax prior to treatment applications.

Extraction

The extraction of open or closed comedones, milia, and pustules is a service that clients expect and need. Extractions must be done very carefully and following strict infection-control guidelines to prevent injury of the skin. Expect extractions to result in skin redness and mild edema, and explain this to the client. The technique employed will vary with individual state guidelines. The use of cold therapy following extraction and soothing, healing agents can minimize this consequence. The client must be prepared for resulting redness and for proper home care afterwards to prevent infection.

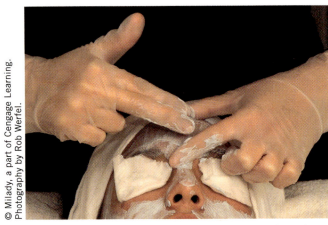

FIGURE 8–4 Manual microdermabrasion is a popular form of exfoliation.

© Milady, a part of Cengage Learning.
Photography by Rob Werfel.

Exfoliation

Exfoliation is the removal of the oldest skin cells on the outermost surface of the skin (Figure 8–4). Many forms of exfoliation are available, including mechanical and chemical methods. The consequences generally associated with exfoliation tend to result from the esthetician's being too aggressive or not properly following manufacturer guidelines. Minimizing consequences begins with proper skin evaluation and a thorough knowledge of the product or equipment being used.

Brushes, scrubs, or any harsh mechanical peeling techniques used in exfoliating treatments generally only cause the desired consequence of mild redness. This can vary based on the client's skin thickness and sensitivity, the amount of pressure used, and the length or duration of the treatment. To prevent a consequence from turning into something more severe, avoid using the exfoliating agent on areas of visible or distended capillaries, thin or sensitive skins, and older skin that bruises easily. It is best to avoid performing aggressive exfoliation treatments on skin that is acne-prone or being medically treated as such. Be cautious of the amount of pressure used and the quality of the brush when using one.

Microdermabrasion

Microdermabrasion is a commonly requested treatment with benefits of smoothing coarse skin and diminishing sun damage, fine lines, and wrinkles. This is achieved by spraying or hand application of high-grade microcrystals. With regard to controlling consequences with microdermabrasion treatments, be aware of the settings used on the device and the number and speed of the passes. When using crystals, the slower the hand moves, the more aggressive the result will be, as more crystals will strike the skin. With diamond tips, the aggression is controlled by the proper selection of the tip and the amount of pressure exerted by the esthetician's hand. Start with the manufacturer's recommended settings for a new client and work your way up based on how the client's skin responds.

During the treatment the client should be consulted to ensure that the level is not uncomfortable. It is normal for the skin to be pink in tone, but the surface should remain intact and without abrasions. The client should be counseled on proper home care and advised not to use peels, scrubs, or anti-aging products with exfoliants in them, nor to have sun exposure following the treatment. A client who does not follow these guidelines could trigger sensitivity, a burn, or

STATE REGULATORY ALERT

Microdermabrasion rules and regulations vary from state to state, so be certain you check legality with your state board.

hyperpigmentation. An esthetician should have proper training and certification prior to offering the advanced-level treatment of microdermabrasion.

Enzymes

Enzymes are a gentle form of exfoliation that is routinely performed with only mild and expected reddening of the skin as a consequence. Common ingredients include papain, derived from papaya, and pancreatin, derived from beef by products; thoroughly discuss client allergies to these as well as other ingredients. Enzymes are reliable and predictable, causing less irritation than physical exfoliation. If they have been blended by the manufacturer to include other acids, the consequences can be greater and the client should be educated accordingly. Other vegetable and fruit resources are also being used for exfoliating enzymes. These should be selected based on the client's skin type and tolerance. Some are very gentle, while others are described as more aggressive.

Some manufacturers provide protocols for buffering meant to reduce the action of enzymes or other exfoliants. Always consider a client's tolerance for a given product and follow the manufacturer recommendations. Having repeat clients is worth more than attempting to meet client demands for powerful treatments and having the treatments go too far and do more harm than good.

Peels

Chemical exfoliation, including the use of alpha hydroxy acids (AHAs) and beta hydroxy acids (BHAs) as well as other acids or acidic blends, is a popular service with clients. Common AHAs and BHAs include glycolic, lactic, malic, tartaric, citric, and salicylic acids. The risks of using these exfoliants are related to the product used, its concentration and pH, and the application techniques for the individual client. Esthetic peels are not true peels but superficial exfoliation. The result is glowing, healthier-looking skin that may be slightly pink following the treatment. Clients should be counseled ahead of time to avoid tanning booths for at least 72 hours prior to and following the treatment. Realistically, a client who routinely uses tanning booths is a poor candidate for chemical exfoliation because of the risk of hyperpigmentation.

If an esthetician desires to offer more aggressive peels, it must be within the scope of practice to do so. It is also recommended that estheticians develop a relationship with a medical professional so they have a place to refer clients should an issue develop. Skin does not always respond to a peel in a predictable manner, and the esthetician should always be prepared for any unexpected consequence.

Some peels will activate an increase in skin cell turnover, which can result in flakiness. Clients must be made aware of this possible consequence. It is critical that they be provided with a healing home-care product designed to be used post-peels and taught how and why to use it. Not using a post-peel product can lead to excess flakiness, irritation, and inflammation or the development of a minor wound. Any time there is a wound; there is a risk of infection and post-inflammatory hyperpigmentation.

If the product contains BHAs, these penetrate into the skin and are flushed from the body via the kidneys. Only the superficial product is removed. If the client engages in vigorous exercise or uses hot showers, saunas, or hot tubs, it can

FYI

Clients should be instructed not to pull or pick at their peeling skin as this can cause serious damage and possible skin pigmentation.

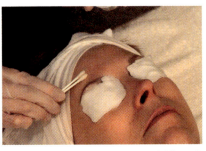

FIGURE 8–5 Always apply a peel thin and evenly and never with an aggressive touch.

trigger the acid to reactivate and stinging and discomfort can again occur as a consequence of the heat and stimulation. Client education and written home-care guidelines can minimize this issue. This type of peel should never be used on a pregnant client.

Proper or improper application of an acid can also minimize or exacerbate consequences. The topical applications should be applied very thinly and evenly. Uneven application, drips, or multiple applications will increase the amount of acid in a particular spot, and the likelihood of red, burned, or injured skin increases (Figure 8–5). This is a consequence of a specific action—over-application of product—and can be avoided with proper training and by carefully following manufacturer's directions. Exfoliation methods should not be combined unless the manufacturer specifically recommendeds it. Most manufacturers advise NOT offering both a chemical peel and microdermabrasion in the same treatment. The risk for problems beyond the expected consequences is significant, and most insurance firms will opt not to cover an insurance claim if manufacturer directions were not followed. It is always important to consider the consequences of redness, flakiness, or irritation and include them as a required component of client education prior to a peel.

Heat

There are many modalities and methods we use to impart heat to the client's skin, including steam, hot towels, hot stones, heated electrical masks or mitts, and heating pads that go under the client to keep them warm. The direct consequence of too much heat is redness and discomfort. It is important to test the method being used to ensure client comfort. Any time you use a heat source, discuss the client's comfort level and adjust the source as needed.

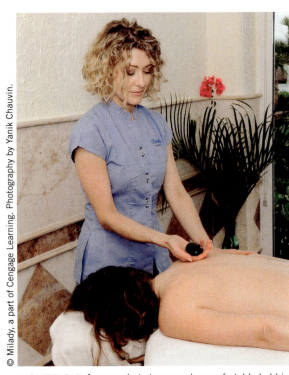

FIGURE 8–6 Assure a hot stone can be comfortably held in the hand before applying on the client.

- Steamers should be placed close enough to generate warmth but not close enough to burn the client.
- Hot towels should be cool enough for the esthetician to hold.
- Hot stones should be able to be held in the hand before applying to the client; the temperature of the stones increases with continued contact (Figure 8–6).
- Electric mitts and masks can develop worn areas and hot spots with use; check them regularly.
- Heating pads should be cozy but not uncomfortably hot.
- Always test hot wax prior to applying it on a client.

Following the application of heat, the skin will appear pink to red, depending on the client's tendency to flush. Adjust to a cooler temperature if the client flushes easily or seems to be uncomfortable.

Claustrophobic Clients

Some people feel fear or genuine discomfort when faced with the sensation of being trapped or closed in. This may extend to wanting a door left open or lights left on, or preferring not to have anything covering the face. Since these fears cannot be controlled, it is important for an esthetician to ask the right questions to determine what will be within the client's comfort zone. A feeling of being uncomfortable or trapped is especially common for clients receiving a body wrap or when the body is covered during a facial. You may leave all or some of the extremities uncovered to give a feeling of freedom of movement. Different clients feel different degrees of anxiety, so if a client indicates a history of claustrophobia on an intake form, it is essential to gently ask questions and obtain more information so the treatment can be performed safely.

Questions to ask may include:

- Does covering your eyes bother you?
- Are tanning goggles better for you than cotton pads as eye protection?
- How do you feel about the use of steam?
- How do you feel about the use of a hot towel wrap?
- What types of masks have you had in past treatments?
- How did you feel about these mask applications?
- Would you be more comfortable if I left more lights on in the room?
- Would you be more comfortable with your arms under or outside the blanket?
- I want to make this quiet and relaxing for you, but would you be more comfortable if I left a door ajar?

Often, clients who perceive themselves as claustrophobic will have far fewer problems in the treatment room than they anticipate. By taking time to address the issue and not ignoring it, we enhance client safety and the treatment outcome.

SIDE EFFECTS OF TREATMENTS

A side effect is a secondary and usually adverse effect, sometimes called a side reaction. It is something that occurs in addition to the intended effect and may be related to drugs, chemicals, or medications. Side effects also include undesirable results that happen in conjunction with an event. Side effects may occur due to medications, allergies, or other unexpected reasons (Figure 8–7).

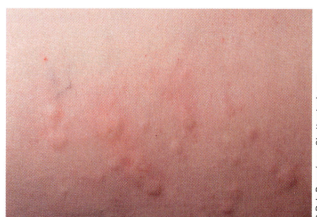

FIGURE 8-7 Irritated skin or a rash is a common side effect of many treatments.

© Rob Byron/www.shutterstock.com

Medications

In the treatment room, a side effect may occur if the client is taking a medication that can have an impact on the skin and the technician is unaware of it. It is crucial to have a thorough discussion of medication during the consultation, but the client may not wish to disclose a medication or simply forget about it. Many medications, both oral and topical, have skin-related side effects, and when they interact with skin treatments, a treatment room issue can result. Unexpected rashes, redness, or irritation may occur immediately or post-treatment. Some medications can trigger this in as little as two weeks, so it is important to check with a client prior to every visit about changes in medications. If in doubt perform a test patch in an inconspicuous area and monitor the results for several minutes before proceeding. If any issues do occur, further treatment should not take place as long as the client is on the medication.

For more details on what to expect from specific medications, please refer to Appendix A in the back of this book.

Allergies

Side effects in our treatment room can also occur when the client's body chemistry is not compatible with the product being used. Allergies can develop at any time, so it is practical to treat every treatment as if it were the first and monitor the skin for results. If using a new product on the client's skin, check the client history form for potential allergies to ingredients in the formula. If a client is allergic to iodine, shellfish, seaweed, or peanuts, then extreme caution should be exercised when considering any product containing seaweed or peanut oil. Follow the guidelines in Chapter 9 (First Aid) for handling an allergic reaction in the clinic.

Burns or Abrasions

Burns or abrasions are undesired results that can happen in conjunction with a treatment. They may be caused by aggressive work on sensitive skin areas, medication-related issues, or a client not following recommended pre- and post-treatment care. They can also be caused by a technician error in judgment. Avoid such errors by completing a thorough, unrushed consultation and providing client education for pre- and post-treatment. When burns or abrasions do unfortunately result, the best plan of action is to follow the first-aid guidelines outlined in Chapter 9. Follow up with the client sincerely by demonstrating a concerned and caring attitude.

Many skin care practices include statements on their informed consent forms that alert clients to the risks of specific treatments. Special risks for Brazilian waxing might include irritation, skin abrasions, or skin tearing. As the groin is an area of concentrated staph and other microorganisms, the risk of infection from these injuries is increased. No injury should ever be ignored, and appropriate action should be taken. Special risks for IPL or laser treatments could include skin irritation, epidermal damage, minor burns, and hypo- or hyperpigmentation. These incidents do happen, so it is important to be prepared and to alert the client to the possibility.

COMPLICATIONS OF TREATMENTS

Complications are defined as issues, factors, or conditions that result unexpectedly in the course of dealing with a condition. It is something that aggravates or complicates a condition and makes things more difficult to treat. A good example would be a wound from a laser hair removal treatment that becomes infected. Laser hair removal may also result in immediate hyperpigmentation (Figure 8–8). In addition, it can actually stimulate hair growth; this is a rare complication and is termed "paradoxical hair growth." Clients with Fitzpatrick IV or darker skin types are generally the only clients who may experience this complication.

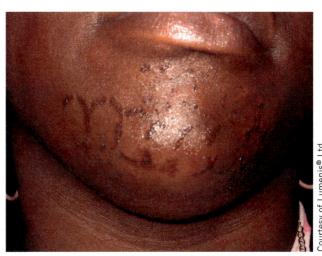

FIGURE 8-8 Hyperpigmentation may result immediately following laser hair removal.

Most complications that occur in the esthetics room are in the first two categories: either consequences or side effects. They are less serious and more easily resolved with good client counseling, informed consent, adherence to manufacturer guidelines, and prudent decision making.

Medical Referrals

Having proper written protocols and post-treatment instructions for every treatment offered is the best method of avoiding complications, but an unexpected situation may occur. Sometimes it is unclear how a situation should be handled. The best guide is to consider the cause and extent of the situation and the amount of damage or trauma to the skin. It is also useful to develop relationships with medical professionals so that if a client comes in requesting a treatment (or a result) that you cannot provide, you will be prepared to offer the appropriate referral (Figure 8–9).

Superficial Redness

In the case of excessive skin redness following a treatment, the esthetician should take appropriate steps to reduce the skin's reaction. Cool compresses or globes, soothing products, and calming light therapies are all helpful methods. If you note signs of minor skin irritation, send the client home with a soothing product and follow up with to make sure that the issue resolves itself. Document the incident in the client's file to avoid repetition.

Breach or Break in the Epidermis

Follow first-aid guidelines for dealing with minor skin injuries. This may include administering a first-aid ointment and bandaging. Discuss how the issue

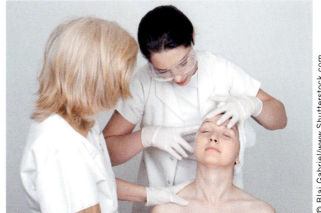

FIGURE 8-9 Develop positive relationships with medical professionals for referral purposes.

should be handled at home with the client and follow up to be sure the issue is resolved. Advise the client to consult a physician should there be signs of swelling or infection. Document the incident in the client's file.

Deeper Wounds or Injuries

Follow first-aid guidelines and get the client appropriate medical care. Assist the client in a caring, concerned manner. Document the incident and provide this information to your insurance carrier if required.

NON-TREATMENT-RELATED INCIDENTS

Some incidents may occur irrespective of the treatment being performed. According to the Equal Employment Opportunity Commission (EEOC), harassment can include "sexual harassment" or unwelcome sexual advances, requests for sexual favors, and other verbal or physical harassment of a sexual nature. In some unfortunate situations, a client, coworker, or employer may be accused of making inappropriate advances to the technician. Take a proactive approach to avoiding this type of situation and inform the harasser that his or her actions are creating an uncomfortable environment for you. If necessary, remove yourself from the situation or request assistance. Always report every incident in writing, even seemingly minor ones, to the business owner or supervisor. If your workplace has established internal grievance policies, be certain to follow the required steps. Seek legal assistance if your concern is not addressed or you feel that legal action is necessary.

Other non-treatment-related incidents may also occur. If a client should faint, have a seizure, or exhibit symptoms of heart attack, stroke, or another illness, call 9-1-1 or follow first-aid guidelines provided in Chapter 9, *First Aid and Emergency Situations*. Stay calm and remain with the client; use the clinic alert system for assistance if necessary.

Prevention of treatment room complications is a key indicator of your safe practices. Be prepared by being educated in product and ingredient usage, know how to maintain and properly use all equipment, and never rush the consultation. Know what action to take if an unfortunate complication arises, and follow up with the client afterwards.

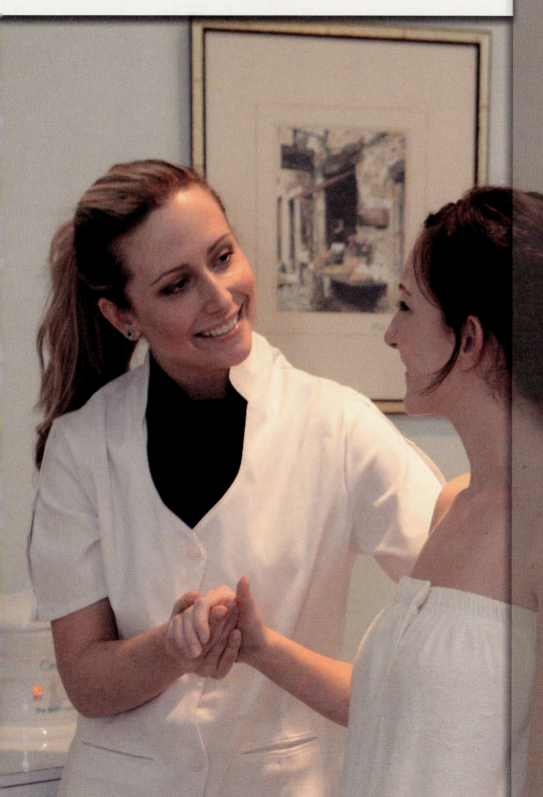

First Aid and Emergency Situations

INTRODUCTION

Regardless of whether we fall under OSHA rules or are exempt from them (a sole practitioner working alone), it only makes good sense to follow the OSHA guidelines to provide protection for ourselves and our clients. An esthetician should establish procedures that will prevent or deter occupational hazards, but also be aware accidents may happen at any time. As licensed professionals, we need to have the first-aid training and supplies commensurate with the hazards that exist in our salons, clinics, and spas. A spa with showers, a pool, and a Vichy shower will present different hazards from a clinic with none of these attributes. More safety protocols would have to be followed where we and the clients are interacting with any form of water modality. A facility that uses electrical modalities like galvanic, high-frequency, microdermabrasion, ultrasonic, laser, or IPL will have uniquely different safety concerns. The details of each workplace safety and first-aid program will depend on its individual circumstances.

DEFINING FIRST AID

First aid refers to care or medical attention that is usually administered immediately after an incident at the location where the injury occurred (Figure 9–1). It is defined as a one-time, short-term treatment that requires little technology or training to administer. The scope of first aid includes cleaning minor cuts, scrapes, or scratches; treating a minor burn; applying bandages or dressings; using over-the-counter medications; draining blisters; flushing the eye; massage; and offering fluids to relieve heat stress.

FIGURE 9–1 The international symbol of First Aid is green and white.

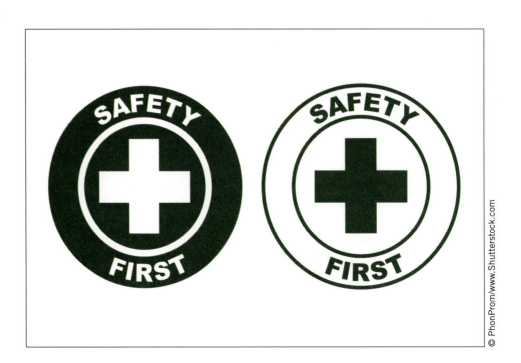

© PhonProm/www.Shutterstock.com

RED CROSS TRAINING

It is recommended that all estheticians, or—even broader—all those in the fields of cosmetology who deal with people of a diverse range of ages on a daily basis, have basic first-aid training. Accidents can happen throughout the spa or salon: slipping on a wet spot, tripping over cords, falls, nicks from sharp implements, burns from hot tools, or injury from products applied to the skin, hair, or body can all occur. In salons that cater to families, it is routinely observed that young children can "find" an accident waiting to happen. Salons and spas tend to have a larger active population of senior citizens, and these clients have special risks and health concerns a professional should be prepared to deal with.

Red Cross first-aid, cardiac pulmonary resuscitation (CPR) and automated external defibrillator (AED) classes are readily available in most towns as well as on-line. Taking these classes will help staff respond to any incident with more confidence and knowledge. The NCEA requires estheticians to take this training, and to maintain their status, if they wish to apply for national certification.

Red Cross Guidelines

Red Cross training provides guidelines for each esthetician or other staff member to follow in case of an accident. In addition, numerous Web sites can be a great resource in the case of a non-emergency medical incident. Having one of these bookmarked or listed as a favorite on your computer can get you quick access to information on treating minor issues and emergency preparedness. You may request or clarify sources of first-aid information from your insurance provider. This will provide you with the peace of mind that you are receiving adequate and accurate information.

Assessment of Care

Your first step in providing care should be to assess the situation. Stop and evaluate before rushing or causing panic. Be practical and use your senses, looking for unusual sights, unusual appearances or behaviors, unusual odors, and unusual noises. Then consider the following:

- Is the scene safe?
- Are there invisible hazards like electricity or poisonous fumes?
- What happened?
- How long ago did it happen?
- Is the situation stable, or could something more happen?
- How many victims are there?
- Can they talk?
- Are they breathing?
- Is there a heartbeat?
- Is there serious bleeding?
- Is there serious pain or the inability to use a body part?

In some situations, it may be hard to recognize an emergency or illness. Ask questions that may help you determine what is wrong.

If you are alone, call 9-1-1 first before attempting to assist. If available, a Bluetooth type of hands-free device or speakerphone will allow you to be on the line with help and to assist the injured person at the same time.

Protect Yourself When Providing First Aid

While you are at low risk of getting infection when offering first aid, you may further minimize risk by following these guidelines:

- Avoid touching bodily fluids if possible.
- Wear skin barrier protection if available (remove your rings or other jewelry that could harbor microorganisms).
- Do not eat, drink, smoke, apply cosmetics or lip balm, handle contact lenses, or touch your eyes, nose, or mouth while your hands or skin may be contaminated.
- Do not handle objects such as pens, clipboard, telephone, or keys while your hands are contaminated.
- Clean up the accident scene, containing, disinfecting, and disposing of contaminants.
- Dispose of contaminated items properly, following OSHA and CDC guidelines.
- Wash hands thoroughly with soap and water after removal.
- Always have a properly equipped first aid kit available.

Before giving first aid to a conscious adult, you must obtain that person's permission to assist him or her. A person has the right to accept or decline your offer. Do not give care to a conscious person who refuses it. To obtain consent, give your name, state that you are trained in first aid, and offer your assistance. Ask the person what he or she thinks may be wrong; if the person cannot tell you, offer your assessment and then explain your plan of action.

Calling for Help

One golden rule is that if you can't decide how severe a condition is, or are unsure of what to do, you should call 9-1-1. The provided list is not all-inclusive, and if you are uncertain whether to call or not, it is best to err on the side of calling emergency services, as the trained professionals may be able to provide more specific direction. Here are some examples of when to call for emergency assistance:

- Unconsciousness
- Trouble breathing or breathing in a strange way
- Not breathing
- No signs of life
- Persistent chest pain
- Severe bleeding that does not stop
- Deep burns to the face and neck
- Pressure or pain in the abdomen that does not go away
- Vomiting blood or passing blood
- Any form of seizure
- Possible head, neck, or back injury
- Apparent poisoning

- Any obvious bone deformity
- Sudden severe headache or slurred speech
- Fire or explosion
- Presence of poisonous gas
- Downed electrical wires
- Swiftly moving or rapidly rising water
- Motor vehicle collision or accident
- Persons who cannot be moved easily

FIRST-AID KIT

The contents of your first-aid kit may vary depending on the type of treatments offered at each facility and the type of accidents that the kit is designed to deal with. Provided below are some general guidelines indicating the items that should be in all first-aid or emergency kits (Figure 9–2).

- Emergency services telephone numbers – 9-1-1
- Addresses of local hospitals
- Poison control number
- Basic first-aid reference cards
- First-aid record of treatment forms
- Emergency reference manual
- Pen and notepad
- Flashlights with extra batteries (small and large)
- Box of non-latex disposable gloves
- 1 pair scissors
- 1 pair tweezers
- 5 safety pins
- Eye-wash supplies
- Breathing barrier with one-way valve
- Oral thermometer (non-mercury, non-glass)
- Disposable thermometer covers
- 5–4″ × 4″ sterile gauze pads
- 5–3″ × 3″ sterile gauze pads
- 5–2″ × 2″ sterile gauze pads

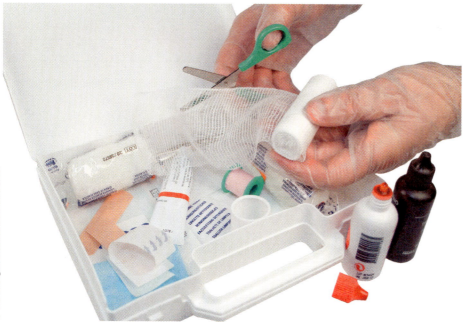

FIGURE 9–2 First-aid kits are necessary to properly deal with minor incidents.

- 2 absorbent compress dressings 5″ × 9″
- 25 adhesive bandages, assorted sizes
- 2 rolls adhesive cloth tape, 10 yds. × 1″
- 2 sterile eye pads
- 2 triangular bandages
- 2–2″ roller bandages
- 2–3″ roller bandages
- 2–4″ roller bandages
- 5 antibiotic ointment packages
- 5 hydrocortisone ointment packets
- 5 burn cream or aloe vera packets
- 5 antiseptic wipe packets
- 4–25 mg Diphenhydramine (oral antihistamine)
- 2 aspirin (81 mg each)
- 1 space blanket
- 2 instant cold compresses

FIRST-AID TREATMENT RECORD

To be completed by the attending first aider.

Patient's Name: _____ Age: _____

Address: _____

City: _____ State: _____ Zip: _____

Date: _____ Time: _____

Incident Location: _____

Emergency Contact: _____ Telephone: _____

Details of Injury:

_____

_____

_____

_____

Significant Medical History:

_____

_____

_____

_____

First Aid Procedures Initiated: (Note Time)

_____:_____

_____

_____:_____

_____

_____:_____

_____

First Aid Provided By: _____

Contact Telephone: _____

The above list and the first-aid responder form courtesy of Susanne Warfield, Paramedical Consultants, Inc. Emergency Medical Care for Your Salon or Spa.

When dealing with an incident that goes beyond minor first-aid care for a staff member or client, the first-aid treatment record should be filled out and a copy retained for at least five years.

COMMON FIRST-AID NEEDS

Basic first-aid training teaches us to deal with the common problems we may encounter. Reviewing the different potential issues will help us to be better prepared. Some of these common problems involve a variety of types of breaks to the skin, allergic reactions, and an assortment of forms of sudden illness. For more serious medical concerns or injuries, first aid will be provided only until medical assistance arrives or is available.

Cuts and Bleeding

Although cuts may be rather rare in a spa or medi-spa setting, they are not uncommon in a salon situation. Stylists routinely work with extremely sharp scissors, and nail technicians can injure the skin with nippers, credo blades, or other sharp devices. The esthetician may need to assist a hairdresser or nail technician in dealing with such an incident. Cuts may also occur during such procedures as difficult extractions or dermaplaning.

When a cut occurs, controlling the bleeding is the first priority. In an injury to the head, the bleeding can be more profuse. Also, clients who are on blood-thinning medications such as aspirin, ibuprofen, or Coumadin® can have more persistent bleeding, even with a minor wound. Any time you need to deal with an injury where there are bodily fluids present, follow standard precautions to prevent the transmission of bloodborne pathogens.

Types of Cuts and Bleeding

A cut to the skin may be minor or deep. Minor cuts are shallow in nature and generally stop bleeding within a few minutes. The wound of a minor cut does not gape open and no underlying dermal tissue, subcutaneous tissue, muscles, or tendons will be visible. Deep cuts often gape open, and underlying tissue may be visible or protrude through the wound. The bleeding of a deeper cut can be generous.

Learn to recognize injury by the type of blood visible:

- Venous blood is dark in color and the bleeding will be steady.
- Capillary blood is bright red in color and is usually involved in a minor or superficial cut.
- Arterial blood is bright red in color and the wound will pulse. It must be treated immediately.

Puncture wounds are less likely to occur in a salon or spa setting. However, if the wound was caused by a dirty or contaminated object, the puncture must be irrigated adequately. For a non-puncture wound, a tetanus shot is not required if the patient has had one in the past 10 years. If there is a puncture wound or another wound that was caused by a dirty or contaminated object, a tetanus booster is recommended if it has been more than five years since a person's last tetanus booster, and depending on the type of wound may be given as a precaution.

Management of Cuts

Minor cuts should have direct pressure applied to control and stop bleeding. Once the bleeding is under control, cleanse the wound with running water and appropriate skin antiseptic. Do not scrub the wound or treat it aggressively. After cleansing, pat dry, apply an antibiotic ointment, and cover with a bandage (Figure 9–3). The client should follow up with a physician in two to three days if needed.

Deep cuts require prompt medical attention and may need stitches. Apply pressure directly to the wound for 20 to 30 minutes using a clean pad or gauze

FIGURE 9–3 The commonly used band aid is available in many styles.

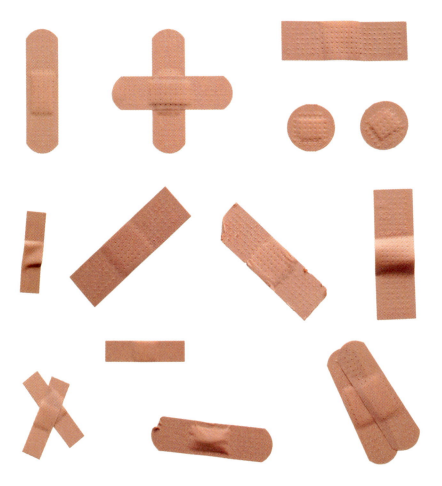

sponge in your gloved hand. Keep the pressure on the wound and resist the temptation to check to see if the bleeding has stopped, as this can trigger more bleeding. If the bleeding stops, the wound can be rinsed and bandaged, and the client may seek medical care. If the bleeding does not slow or is cause for alarm, seek medical assistance or call 9-1-1.

If the wound is on the hand, refer the client for medical attention. Trivial cuts over joints can easily become infected, leading to permanent damage. Even superficial cuts on the hand may require stitches to keep the edges together. People with chronic medical conditions or compromised immune systems are especially at risk. Medical evaluation of hand wounds is always recommended.

Allergic Reactions

Many things can trigger an allergic reaction, the possibility of which can be diminished by conducting a thorough client consultation. However, allergic reactions may occur unexpectedly at any time. A client may do fine with a skin-care product for years and then develop sensitivity to it. Medications, compromised immune systems, and health conditions contribute to sensitivities and allergic reactions. Reactions may take place immediately or can take hours to develop.

FYI

Asthma is commonly related to allergies, and thorough client consultation should provide clues to potential irritants and help the technician develop an individual treatment plan.

Localized Allergic Reactions

A localized allergic reaction may manifest with localized redness, rashes, hives, or itching. Remove the offending substance, rinse thoroughly, and apply cold compresses. Once the skin has calmed, cleanse with a mild cleanser and apply an over-the-counter hydrocortisone product to the area. While estheticians cannot administer oral drugs, even over-the-counter ones, we may suggest the client take an antihistamine if the client desires. Some people may become very agitated from taking an antihistamine, while others become very sleepy. Clients who are uncertain of their bodies' reaction to oral antihistamines should not drive.

Anaphylaxis

Anaphylaxis is the most serious type of allergic reaction. Call 9-1-1 immediately, as it is life-threatening and can progress rapidly. Symptoms include confusion, anxiety, unconsciousness, nausea, vomiting, abdominal pain, swelling of the tongue or lips, and difficulty breathing. A person experiencing an anaphylactic response may be pale or exhibit a red rash, hives, or itching. A client with a history of anaphylaxis may carry an EpiPen injector or inhaler to dilate lung airways. Request the client's permission to assist with obtaining and administering the medication.

After calling 9-1-1, help the client be comfortable and loosen tight-fitting clothing. Turn the client on his or her side so that there is no risk of choking if the client vomits. If the client is unconscious and/or is not breathing, perform CPR until help can take over.

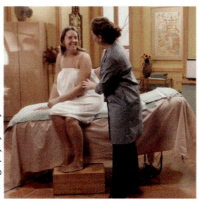

FIGURE 9–4 Always assist clients if they are feeling weak.

Fainting

Fainting is the loss of consciousness caused by a decrease in the blood supply to the brain. Fainting may occur spontaneously and without any warning. Prior to the incident, the client may feel lightheaded or notice tunnel or blurred vision. Most causes of fainting are not serious, but until the cause can be determined, it must be treated as a serious situation. Any fainting episode may be triggered by an underlying medical condition such as a heart condition or seizure. Other causes of fainting could be as simple as emotional stress triggered by anxiety or a defense mechanism of the human body when rebounding from a stressful situation. Heart rhythm abnormalities, medication usage, diabetes, heart disease, and seizure disorders can all trigger fainting. If a client faints, you should require that the client seek medical evaluation and obtain a physician's release before agreeing to perform further treatments.

To treat a fainting episode, help a lightheaded client to a chair (Figure 9–4). Encourage the client to lie flat and elevate the legs above the heart. Loosen tight or restrictive clothing, especially in the neck and waist areas. Check for pulse and heart rate and note whether the rate is steady or irregular. If the heartbeat is irregular or if the individual does not immediately regain consciousness, call 9-1-1.

If consciousness is regained, assess the client's condition by addressing him or her in accelerating tones and noting the response.

If a person regains consciousness from a faint, ask:

- What is your name?
- Do you know where you are?
- What is the date and time?

Those suffering from a simple fainting episode will revive quickly and be able to answer these questions. Ask about symptoms such as shortness of breath, chest pain, abdominal pain, headache, weakness, and numbness. Unless the cause of the episode is clear, medical evaluation is necessary. Arrange for transport to the nearest emergency room or urgent care facility for evaluation. If the cause is clear, encourage the client to lie down for 15 to 20 minutes before allowing him or her to get up or leave. It is a good idea to arrange transportation and not allow the client to drive.

Shock

Shock is a life-threatening condition that occurs when the body is not getting enough blood flow. Shock can cause damage to multiple organs very quickly. The condition requires immediate medical treatment and can progress at a rapid pace. Shock may result from trauma, allergic reactions, heatstroke, or other causes.

Common symptoms of shock may include:

- Skin is cool and clammy to the touch.
- Skin appears pale or gray.
- Pulse is weak and rapid.
- Breathing may be slow and shallow or rapid.

- Blood pressure is below normal.
- Pupils may be dilated, lacking luster, staring.
- Person may be conscious or unconscious.
- Person may feel faint, weak, or confused.
- Person may be overly excited and anxious.

If you suspect shock, call 9-1-1 and follow directions until assistance arrives. If the person is conscious and there is no evidence of injury to the head, neck, legs, or spine, assist the person in lying down. Check the airway, breathing, and circulation. Keep the person from moving unnecessarily, loosen tight clothing, and keep make sure the person is warm and comfortable. If the person vomits or drools from the mouth, turn the head to the side to prevent choking, as long as there is no chance of spinal injury. Stay with the person until emergency medical services arrive.

Burns

The skin is designed to protect the underlying organs; skin is a barrier of protection from external elements and microorganisms. The skin has many defense mechanisms and also provides sensation so that we can respond to the world around us. Burns can affect the epidermis as a superficial wound or extend deeper into the dermis or below. The depth of the burn is directly related to the extent of the injury and the classification of the burn. Burns can be caused by thermal (heat) sources, chemicals, electricity, or radiation. Burn treatment will depend on the cause, degree, and location of the burn.

Burns occur in varying amounts of damage and skin depth. These can be classified into three degrees, as outlined here (Figure 9–5):

- First-degree burns have redness, swelling, and possible pain; these only affect the epidermis.
- Second-degree burns exhibit the above signs with the addition of intense redness and blisters; this type of burn has reached the deeper dermal layer of the skin.
- Third-degree burns affect all layers of the skin and may involve underlying muscles, fat, bones, and nerves. Affected skin may be dry and white or charred in appearance. This type of burn may be extremely painful or numb and will result in permanent damage.

Treatment of Thermal Burns

Thermal burns generally occur when contact is made with any heat source that is higher than the body temperature. Many items in esthetic treatments can cause this to occur. The causes of thermal burns may range from heated towels, wax, stones, or hot water to directly from electrical sources. Always practice safe testing for each item that could lead to a potential burn.

First-Degree Thermal Burns   These are also called superficial burns and only affect the epidermis or surface of the skin. The skin will appear red and dry and is usually tender and painful. Cool the burn with cool running water or cool compresses until the pain is relieved. Do not use ice or apply icepacks, as this can cause frostbite to the tissue. Apply burn or antibiotic ointment to the area and

CAUTION

Persons who are in shock often complain of severe thirst. Never give a person in shock anything by mouth, including offering anything to eat or drink!

HERE'S A TIP

The first step in burn management is to check the scene for safety, then remove or stop the source of the burn. Once the source has been eliminated or removed, progress with burn treatment.

CAUTION

Third-degree burns are always a medical emergency. Immediately call 9-1-1!

First-Degree Burn

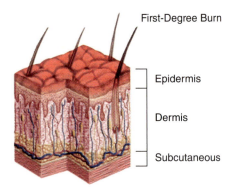

Epidermis

Dermis

Subcutaneous

Second-Degree Burn

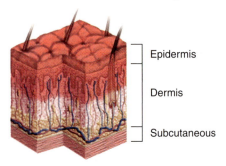

Epidermis

Dermis

Subcutaneous

Third-Degree Burn

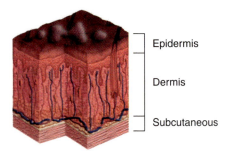

Epidermis

Dermis

Subcutaneous

Fourth-Degree Burn

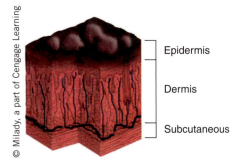

Epidermis

Dermis

Subcutaneous

© Milady, a part of Cengage Learning

FIGURE 9–5 Three degrees of burns.

cover the burn loosely with a sterile dressing. Most first-degree burns will not require further attention. But if the burn covers a large area or an esthetic area such as the face, or if it involves hands, feet, groin, buttocks, or a major joint, it should be evaluated by a medical professional.

Second-Degree Thermal Burns   Second-degree burns are sometimes called partial thickness burns and involve the top layers of the skin. The skin will be red, usually painful, have blisters that may open, and weep clear fluid; the skin may appear mottled and it often swells. These burns can take three to four weeks to heal and may leave scars. If they are less than 3 inches square and do not involve the critical areas mentioned under first-degree burns, treat as a minor burn. Cool the skin using cold water or compresses; follow this with the application of burn or antibiotic ointment. Cover loosely with a clean, sterile gauze or bandage. Over-the-counter pain medication may be taken to reduce discomfort. Always leave any blisters intact. For any second-degree burns that exceed 3 square inches, or that involve face, hands, feet, or joints, have the burn promptly evaluated by a medical professional.

Third-Degree Thermal Burns   Third-degree burns are a medical emergency and you should immediately call for emergency medical services. The skin affected by a third-degree burn will appear white and leathery and may be painless. Ensure that the client's clothing is not smoldering, but do not attempt to remove burnt clothing. If possible, elevate the burned body part or parts above the heart and cover large burn areas with a clean, dry sterile cloth or bandages. Do not use cold water or moist sheets over large areas, as this could induce hypothermia. Until assistance arrives, monitor breathing and circulation and perform CPR if necessary.

Electrical Shock and Burns   The degree of the shock or burn that a victim may suffer depends on the electrical current the person was exposed to. There may be no visible signs of injury, as in the case of low-voltage injuries, or there may be significant tissue destruction. A small burn mark is a common symptom, but the extent of damage may be much greater.

   With alternating current (AC), the current causes a continuous contracting of the muscles the current is flowing through. It is the amperage of the current rather than the voltage that can trigger irregular heartbeat or sudden death due to the impact on the heart. The high-frequency unit used in a spa or salon does not cause muscle contraction. Other devices used for muscle contraction are outside the scope of practice for licensed estheticians in most states.

   Direct-current (DC) injuries tend to be associated with high-voltage sources. While the current is shorter, the tissue damage escalates with increasing voltage. Galvanic devices should be used with care and attention given to precautions and contraindications.

The path of the current also determines potential injury. Hand-to-hand and hand-to-foot current flow travels through the heart and spinal cord and so tends to be the most damaging. The type of tissue involved in electrical current flow also affects the degree of the damage. Fat, bone, and tendons have high resistance, resulting in more heat for an electrical current and possibly causing greater tissue destruction.

Treat electrical contact by first shutting off the power source at the circuit breaker panel. Do not attempt to shut off the power at the device that the victim is in contact with. Next, remove the client from the power source. Check for signs of breathing and a pulse; if necessary, begin CPR and call 9-1-1. Only if the victim is conscious, offer care for shock and thermal burns. Any person who has been exposed to electrical shock should be evaluated by a medical professional.

CAUTION

Never go near someone with an electrical burn until you are sure the person is no longer in contact with the power source.

Chemical Burns

Most chemicals that can burn the skin are either a strong acid or strong alkaline. In the spa, medi-spa, or salon, these high- or low-pH products are found in the form of the chemicals used in professional treatments. Chemical burns most frequently occur on the face, eyes, hands, and arms. Most chemical burns are minor and require minimal care. The degree of the burn is determined by the type of chemical, the strength or pH of the chemical, the quantity of the chemical, and the duration of exposure. If the chemical came into direct contact with the eyes or other mucous membrane, the injury can be much more severe.

A mild chemical burn will cause redness and irritation with occasional blisters. Flush the area with cool water for at least 20 minutes. If the chemical is a powder, brush off the powder before rinsing with water. If burning persists, flush with running water for 20 minutes. Apply antibiotic or medicated ointment, cover with sterile loose gauze or a bandage, and refer the person to a physician.

If the chemical was inhaled, respiratory track irritation or burns can occur, resulting in coughing, sore throat, shortness of breath, and wheezing. In this situation, the victim should receive a medical evaluation. If the person suffered chemical burns over a large surface area, is dizzy or pale, or has chest pain, shortness of breath, difficulty breathing, or eye injury, seek immediate medical evaluation.

CAUTION

All physical or chemical burns on the face, groin, hands, and feet and second-degree chemical burns larger than three inches should be evaluated by a medical professional.

Eye Injuries

Eye injuries may occur when any form of irritant—either a foreign body or product—enters the eye. Injuries are often minor but some could cause temporary or permanent loss of vision. In the esthetics setting, eye injuries can be a result of foreign bodies getting into the eye, corneal abrasions, or chemical burns (Figure 9–6). The risk of eye injury may be less than that of eye irritation, but the possibility still exists of a cut or abrasion to the cornea or other portion of the eye. In the case of any eye injury, the injured person should remove any contact lenses, since leaving lenses in can increase the risk of eye trauma or damage.

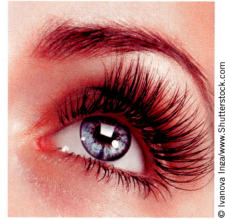

FIGURE 9–6 Always work cautiously around the fragile eye area to prevent an injury.

© Ivanova Inga/www.Shutterstock.com

Corneal Abrasion

A corneal abrasion is a scratch on the cornea, the clear portion of the eye. It may be caused by direct trauma to the cornea via an object such as a fingernail or mascara wand, or from microdermabrasion crystals. If the object becomes lodged under the eyelid, every blink can increase the amount of damage. Corneal abrasions are very painful and cause tearing and redness of the eye, sensitivity to light, and even blurry vision. Flush the eye profusely using an eyewash station or by holding the eye under running tap water. If the foreign body is visible, use a damp cotton swab to assist with removal. Sometimes, blinking can assist removal. Gently cover the eyes or provide dark sunglasses to assist with light sensitivity. Instruct the client to keep fingers away from the eyes and avoid rubbing the area. Assist the client to a place that can provide a medical evaluation.

Foreign Body

A foreign body in the eye may be something as natural as an eyelash, a cotton fiber, or substance from an exfoliation product. The nature of the object and how the accident occurred may determine whether the particle will become embedded or if it can be washed away.

A corneal foreign body occurs when an object such as wood, metal, or plastic becomes embedded in the eye. Symptoms include severe pain, redness, and tearing. If the object is lodged, the person can feel it as he or she blinks and will likely experience blurriness of vision. Refer the person to a medical professional for evaluation. Bleeding in any portion of the eye or a layer of blood behind the cornea indicate a more severe injury. Be aware that the eyes blink together, so close and cover both eyes as you assist the person to a place where treatment can be administered.

In some high-velocity injuries, a foreign body penetrates through and into the eye. Any penetration of the eye by a foreign body must be treated as a medical emergency. Avoid placing pressure on any part of the eyeball that appears to have been cut. Protect an injured eye by covering it appropriately while seeking medical treatment. To treat loose or small foreign bodies, gently flush the eye at an eye-wash station or under running tap water. Hold the eye open to facilitate the flushing. If the object is under the upper eyelid, have the person look down. If under the lower lid, have the person look up. If the object can be seen floating, use a wet cotton swab but do not run the swab across the cornea.

If there is any persistent feeling of a foreign body in the eye, if there is persistent pain or tearing, or if there is blood or clear fluid coming from the eye, the person should be seen by a medical professional. Arrange for the client to be transported for medical assistance if necessary, as an eye injury may result in decreased capacity of vision.

CAUTION

Do NOT attempt to remove any foreign bodies from the eye if they appear embedded. The foreign body could cause a deeper or more severe wound by the slightest movement. Promptly assist the person to a medical facility.

Chemical Eye Injuries

Chemical that enter the eye may lead to irritation or a chemical burn. Irritation is more common, but some chemical burns can cause severe injury or damage to the eye. Every chemical exposure should be taken very seriously. Evaluate what the chemical is and how long the exposure lasted. If taking the client to a medical professional for evaluation, take the offending substance and the Material Safety Data Sheet on it with you.

Chemical burns can be divided into categories based on the substance involved. These can be alkaline, acidic, or irritants. On the potential hydrogen (pH) scale, the eye is close to neutral at approximately 7.4. Alkaline chemicals have a pH above 7 and acid chemicals have a pH below 7. The further the pH of a substance is from the neutral range of 7, the more the strength of the substance intensifies.

Alkaline chemicals can penetrate deep into the cornea and can cause severe damage. Treat them as a medical emergency. Substances with high alkaline properties include drain cleaners, ammonia, sodium, potassium, and calcium hydroxides. These are commonly found in some hair products, depilatories, and powerful cleaning agents.

Chemical burns from an acidic substance are generally less severe than alkaline burns. In esthetic clinics, they would be found in chemical peels such as lactic, glycolic, and trichloroacetic acids (often referred to as TCAs). In a salon environment, many hair and nail products are of an acid-level pH, such as ammonium thioglycolate–based permanent waving solutions or acrylic nail primers.

Chemical irritants are generally the least severe, causing irritation and redness but no damage. These are products with a more neutral pH, such as mild cleansers and toners. All chemical eye injuries may result in redness, tearing, irritation, sensitivity to light, and inability to keep the eye open. Swelling of the white portion of the eye or of the eyelid may occur. Vision may become blurry, but loss of vision will indicate a more severe burn.

All exposure to chemicals in the eye should be treated by flushing the eye with running water or at an eye-wash station for 10 to 20 minutes. Attempt to flush under the eyelids as well to remove the offending substance. If the chemical exposure is a significant acid or alkaline burn, call 9-1-1 and continue flushing the eye. The EMS staff can continue flushing the eye during transit to the medical facility.

Even with a minor irritant, if the discomfort does not improve or if vision changes, the injured person should be seen by a medical professional immediately.

Sudden Illness

Sudden illness is something that occurs unexpectedly and without warning. Quick recognition of sudden illness can greatly assist the person. A client who suddenly looks or feels ill may request that a treatment be discontinued. You should take a few moments and ask some questions, as the client's condition may change rapidly and turn into a life-threatening situation. Discussed above are the topics of fainting and allergic reactions; be aware the client could also be suffering from a diabetic emergency, seizure, poisoning, or heart issues.

Symptoms to watch out for that could indicate the need for medical intervention include the following:

- Nausea or need to vomit
- Blurry vision or loss of vision
- Difficulty speaking or slurred speech
- Numbness and weakness
- Severe headache
- Sweating, pale and ashen skin color

- Skin flushed, dry, warm
- Change in the breathing rate (faster or slower)
- Change in pulse rate
- Persistent chest pressure or pain

Care for Sudden Illness

If you cannot see any apparent reason for a sudden illness, check the person and call 9-1-1 for life-threatening conditions. If the client is attempting to reach medication, this may be a clue to an underlying problem. Stay with the person, monitoring breathing and keeping the person at a comfortable temperature. Provide comfort and reassurance and help the person into the most comfortable position. If a person loses consciousness, monitor breathing and pulse. Stay with the person and make sure the airways remain free until Emergency Medical Services (EMS) can arrive.

Diabetic Emergency

If you determine from responses to the questions you ask that the person is having a diabetic emergency and can safely swallow foods or fluids, it is all right to offer a glucose tablet or other source of sugar, preferably in a liquid form. Good sources include fruit juice, non-diet soda, or a teaspoon of real sugar in water. Assist in completing a glucose check if the client has a monitoring system. If the diabetic carries medication, assist in finding it. If there is no improvement within 5 minutes, call 9-1-1. If the client faints or becomes unresponsive, he or she may be progressing into insulin shock or a diabetic coma. Call 9-1-1 immediately.

Seizures

A seizure may or may not be easy to recognize. There are a wide variety of possible symptoms of seizures, depending what parts of the brain are involved. Many, if not all, types of seizures cause loss of awareness and some cause twitching or shaking of the body.

Some seizures can be challenging to recognize because their symptoms consist of nothing more than a staring spell. Occasionally, seizures can cause temporary changes in sensation or vision. Some forms of seizures result in mild twitching of muscles or more severe convulsions.

If a person is having a seizure, do NOT insert any object into the mouth for him or her to bite on. Instead, protect the person from injury by removing objects that could hurt him or her. Protect the head by placing a soft cushion under or around it. If the person start to vomit or saliva shows around the mouth, roll the person onto his or her side to prevent choking.

Most seizures are brief, and once the seizure is over, normal breathing usually resumes. Offer reassurance and comfort while the person become reoriented. If this occurs in a public space, ask those around you to provide room and allow the person to rest until he or she feels well enough to sit up or move. Medical care should be sought promptly.

Cardiac Emergencies

Cardiac emergencies should always be taken seriously, and if there is any doubt about what is triggering the situation, 9-1-1 should be called. Do not let the victim talk you out of calling for assistance or delaying a call for longer than two minutes. Learn to recognize cardiac emergencies and respond appropriately, as occurrence is possible in any venue at any time.

Cardiopulmonary Resuscitation

Cardiopulmonary resuscitation (CPR) is a combination of rescue breathing and chest compressions delivered to victims thought to be in cardiac arrest. When cardiac arrest occurs, the heart stops pumping blood. CPR can offer circulation and oxygenation to the vital organs until EMS arrives. CPR must begin immediately upon recognition of cardiac arrest to be beneficial.

CPR is administered by providing rapid chest compressions and artificial respirations. Specific methods must be employed to prevent a worsening of the situation. CPR methods vary based on the age of the victim and the situation, so receiving proper training is crucial.

Proper training for the administration of CPR is available from many local agencies. Check with your local Red Cross or any health care provider for information about class enrollment. The training is not difficult and will be beneficial to anyone who participates; no one is exempt from being in a situation where CPR may be needed.

Automated External Defibrillator (AED)

The automated external defibrillator (AED) device is about the size of a laptop computer and is often portable (Figure 9–7). It analyzes the heart's rhythm for any abnormalities and, if necessary, directs the rescuer to deliver an electrical shock to the victim. This shock, referred to as defibrillation, may help to reestablish the heartbeat closer to its natural rhythm. AED devices are easy to operate using voice prompts that instruct the user in exactly what to do.

AEDs in the workplace can reduce treatment time and increase survival odds because they can be used before the emergency team arrives. Employees or clients may suffer a cardiac arrest, and having the AED on-site allows for quick and easy access. Place the AED with the first-aid kit so that response can be within three to five minutes. A centrally accessible area is ideal.

Sudden Cardiac Arrest

Sudden cardiac arrest (SCA) is a leading cause of death in the United States. Sudden cardiac arrest occurs without warning. Many cases are due to abnormal heart rhythms, also called arrhythmias. The majority of these are ventricular fibrillation, a condition in which the electrical impulses of the heart become chaotic. This causes the heart to pump blood ineffectively. Symptoms may include chest or upper

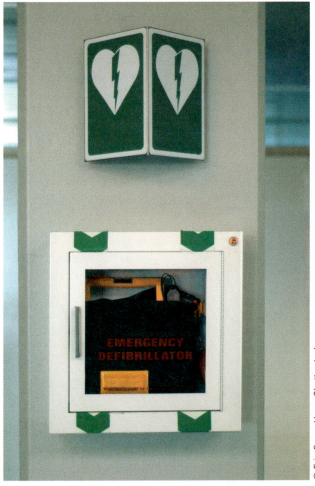

© Eric Gevaert/www.Shutterstock.com

FIGURE 9–7 Emergency defibrillators are becoming more common to many workplaces.

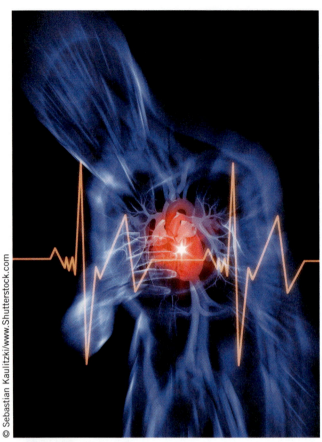

FIGURE 9–8 Sudden cardiac arrest is a leading cause of death in the United States.

body discomfort, shortness of breath, nausea, or lightheadedness. Victims of SCA may collapse and quickly lose consciousness without warning. Death will follow unless a normal heart rhythm is restored; use of an automated external defibrillator (AED) is the best method to improve survival outcomes ("Sudden deaths from Cardiac Arrests," 2004). A busy clinic or spa may want to consider adding an AED device. They can be obtained for as little as $100 for a home-style unit.

Symptoms   It is important to know the symptoms for a cardiac crisis, which may differ slightly from person to person and among men and women (Figure 9–8). Women are just as vulnerable as men to heart attack and account for nearly 50 percent of all heart attack deaths.

General symptoms of a heart attack include the following:

- Chest discomfort: pressure, fullness, squeezing, pain
- Pain or discomfort that extends to one or both arms, the back, the neck, the jaw, or the stomach
- Shortness of breath (with or without chest pain)
- Symptoms of a heart attack more commonly noticed by women include:
  - Breaking out in cold sweat
  - Nausea or vomiting
  - Lightheadedness

Care   If you suspect that your client or coworker is suffering from heart attack symptoms, call 9-1-1 immediately. Be sure to accurately describe the symptoms to the 9-1-1 specialist. This will ensure a priority dispatch of EMS technicians trained in cardiac life support. If the person is awake, have him or her chew a regular-strength aspirin to help inhibit blood clotting. Be sure to tell the EMS technicians that you have done this. If the person is in cardiac arrest and an AED is available, follow the directions and if necessary administer CPR until EMS arrives.

Sudden Cardiac Death

Sudden cardiac death, or death from cardiac arrest, is the abrupt and complete loss of heart function. Cardiac death can occur whether or not a person has been diagnosed with heart disease. Severe cardiac arrest is unexpected, and death can occur instantly or shortly after symptoms appear.

Heart disease is the number one cause of death in the United States. About 50 percent of all deaths related to coronary heart disease are sudden and

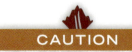

CAUTION

Minutes matter! Never delay more than two minutes to call 9-1-1 for EMS assistance.

unexpected, regardless of the underlying heart problem. Causes of heart disease include clogged arteries, degeneration of the heart muscle, heart enlargement due to high blood pressure, and atherosclerosis. Atherosclerosis is the narrowing of major coronary arteries, scarring from a prior heart attack, thickening of the heart muscle, and arrhythmias. Heart disease is often unrecognized and is a common problem. Heart disease is responsible for the deaths of approximately 1 out of every 4 adults in the United States each year.

Stroke

Stroke is the third cause of death in the United States. A history of high blood pressure (revealed on clients' medical history forms) is an indicator for heightened risk of emergency situations, including stroke, heart attack, heart failure, or kidney failure. Today, many treatments can reduce the risk of damage from the most common types of stroke, but they must be administered in the first three hours. It is crucial to learn to recognize the signs of a stroke.

Warning signs a stroke is occurring appear suddenly and include the following:

- Weakness or numbness of the face, arm, or leg, especially on one side of the body
- Confusion, trouble speaking or understanding
- Trouble seeing in one or both eyes
- Trouble walking, dizziness, loss of balance or coordination
- Severe headache with no known cause

Women often have symptoms unique to females and may also experience the following symptoms, which appear suddenly:

- Face or limb pain
- Hiccoughs
- Nausea
- General weakness
- Chest pain
- Shortness of breath
- Palpitations

Care for Stroke   If you think a person may be exhibiting symptoms of a stroke, follow the recommendations of the National Stroke Association. Any time a person exhibits any symptoms of stroke, call 9-1-1 immediately. Note the time when the symptoms first occurred so that you can inform the EMS team. A special clot-busting medication administered within the first three hours of symptom onset can minimize damage. The National Stroke Association developed the Act F.A.S.T. system of stroke identification; F.A.S.T. is an acronym that stands for Face, Arms, Speech, and Time. This Act F.A.S.T. system involves questions to ask a possible victim, which are listed here:

- **Face:** Ask the person to smile. Does one side of the face droop?
- **Arms:** Ask the person to raise both arms. Does one arm drift downward?

FYI

Recreational drug abuse has been determined to be a cause of sudden cardiac death (SCD).

HERE'S A TIP

Quick action for stroke victims is crucial, as the sooner treatment is administered, the better the chance that permanent damage may be lessened.

- **Speech:** Ask the person to repeat a simple phrase. Are the words slurred or strange? Can the person repeat the sentence correctly?
- **Time:** Call 9-1-1 immediately if any of the symptoms are observed and provide the time of the initial observation.

Transient Ischemic Attack

A transient ischemic attack (TIA) is a "mini-stroke" or "warning stroke." It produces stroke-like symptoms but there is no lasting damage. The only difference between a stroke and a TIA is that the TIA is very temporary; most last less than 5 minutes, with the average only being about one minute. It is important that these be recognized and treated to prevent a stroke from occurring. The American Stroke Association, a division of the American Heart Association, says a TIA should be handled in the same way as a stroke: by calling 9-1-1 and describing the symptoms and when the symptoms began.

Being able to recognize medical situations and knowing the appropriate first aid to administer will protect your staff and your guests (Figure 9–9). Consider using injury-control modules offered by the American Red Cross to make your staff more aware and minimize at-the-clinic injuries.

Seeking the proper education and training is part of your professional responsibilities. Your education and preparedness to administer basic first aid and deal with emergency situations will reduce panic and increase your ability to offer the best possible care.

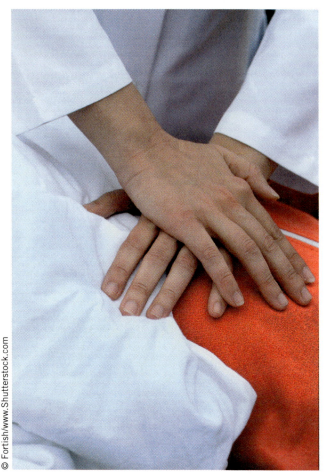

© Fortish/www.Shutterstock.com

FIGURE 9–9 CPR training is available from many local agencies.

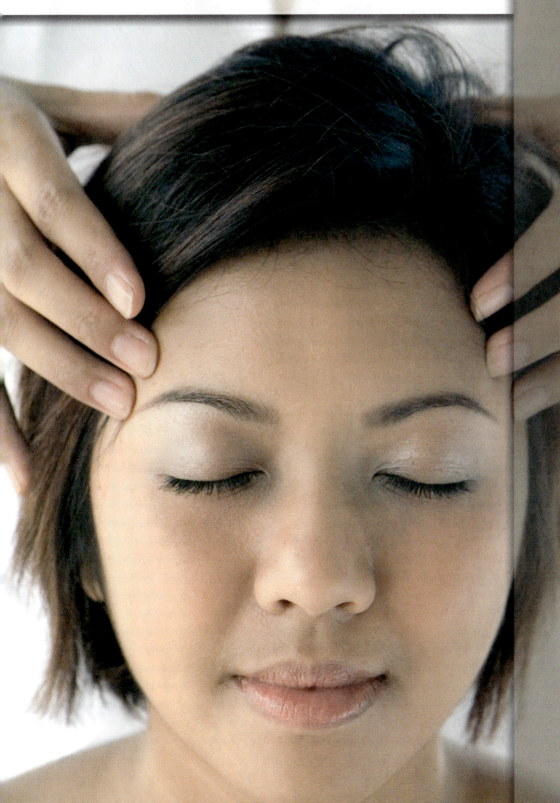

CHAPTER 10

Nutrition, Wellness, and Stress Management

INTRODUCTION

The professional practice of being an esthetician ventures beyond providing treatments for the skin. Clients will often seek your advice on what they can do to improve the appearance and health of their skin. Even though you may inform them of how to properly cleanse and care for their skin, maximum benefits will come from wellness and proper nutrition. The skin is an excellent indicator of overall health and well-being; poor health is commonly represented in the appearance of the skin. The condition, coloration, and appearance of the skin provide clues of genetic ancestry, nutrient intake, lifestyle, and stress levels.

GOOD HEALTH DEALS WITH THE WHOLE PERSON

Numerous factors contribute to the general health and wellness of the human body. These include healthy living and proper nutrition, along with mental and physical fitness. Given the varying views on how best to maintain health and wellness, each person must determine a personal preference to achieve the maximum benefit.

Body, Mind, and Spirit

Overall wellness results from the balance of body, mind, and spirit. When any single aspect is not on an equal footing with the others, negative health issues begin to arise. For example, a poor mental attitude can begin to affect sleep patterns, leading to a general feeling of malaise. If a person does not get enough exercise, the cells of the body do not reaching their maximum capabilities and will result in weakness and fatigue.

Practice proper nutrition and work at getting sufficient physical exercise to maximize your physical health. Always make an effort to receive adequate rest and time to relax to stimulate mental health. Making time to enjoy life will benefit your personal spirit.

Estheticians tend to link components of health care with beauty treatments. Historically, views of health care have differed greatly, as seen in the divide between Eastern philosophy and the practice of Western medicine. In a spa environment, clients expect to see aspects of healthy living, practice of personal health care, and well-being. For this reason, it is important to be familiar with the differences between Eastern and Western medical practices.

REGULATORY AGENCY ALERT

Estheticians may wish to offer clients information regarding medical treatments or practices. Remember, it is not within the scope of practice for an esthetician to give medical advice; be prepared in advance to provide the appropriate referrals.

Eastern Philosophy of Medicine

Fundamental to Eastern philosophy and the practice of traditional Chinese medicine is the belief that the development of wisdom is development of health, and that a healthy life is the perfect balance of mind and body. The Eastern philosophy of true health means that the entire person must be considered and mere treatment of the symptoms is not sufficient. The beliefs of Eastern philosophy are based on notions of energy and the use of nature in the health and wellness of humans.

Some of the more common Eastern philosophies include the beliefs of the yin and the yang, as well as ayurveda and the three dosha principles. The yin and yang are two interacting energies that must work cohesively to achieve balance. Ayurveda means "the science of life" and is a study of longevity or knowing how to live, be well, and manifest one's own natural beauty. The three dosha principles are unique combinations of five universal elements: space, air, earth, fire, and water (Figure 10–1).

Practitioners of Eastern philosophy realize that the internal components of humans are affected by external factors and develop treatment plans accordingly. The practice of treating the person as a whole rather than as an assortment of parts has also been found in the history of Egyptian, Greek, and Roman health care.

Eastern Philosophies   Eastern philosophies use the following to help evaluate the patient:

- Client data
- Client evaluation
- **Doshas:** vata, pitta, kapha
- **Five elements:** space, fire, air, water, earth
- Yin and yang

Ayurveda, or the science of life, uses both the three doshas and the five contributing elements to identify client needs. This includes the belief that an individual has a distinct pattern of energy in a specific combination of physical, mental, and emotional characteristics. The three doshas are the vata, the pitta, and the kapha; each contains varying degrees of dominance of the five elements of space, fire, air, water, and earth. When these characteristics are out of balance, health problems may result. Here are some common examples of energy sources, symptoms, and effects of imbalance:

- Space—cold skin or cold hands and feet; excess = osteoporosis
- Air—fidgety client who has trouble settling down; excess = dryness, flakiness
- Fire—client whose skin flares up easily; excess = redness, inflammation
- Water—client with soft, moist skin; excess = puffiness, edema
- Earth—client with firm skin that ages well; excess = cellulite

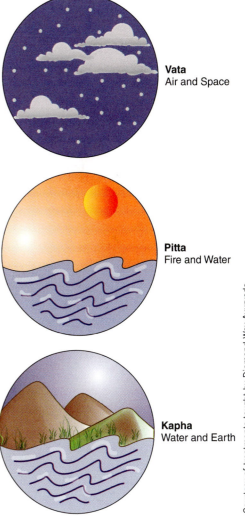

Vata
Air and Space

Pitta
Fire and Water

Kapha
Water and Earth

FIGURE 10–1 Symbols of the three doshas which are combinations of the five elements.

Courtesy of treatments taught by Diamond Way Ayurveda.

- Vata—thin skin, fine pores, drier skin, energetic, multi-tasker
- Pitta—warm skin, T-zone issues, blushes easily, appearance-conscious
- Kapha—cool, oily, thick skin; soft-spoken; grounded; loves routine

Eastern Treatments Once the needs have been established, common Eastern treatment techniques include use of one or more of the following:

- Herbs (oral and/or topical, raw and unprocessed)
- Incense or burning/steaming of herbs
- Oils, botanicals, and essences
- The senses: sight, sound, aroma, touch, taste, and heart feelings (Figure 10–2)
- Temperature of room and treatments
- Reiki
- Color
- Chakra stones
- Massage
- Yoga
- Other relaxation therapies, including meditation or meditative states

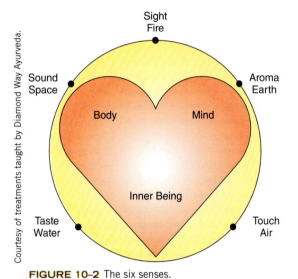

Courtesy of treatments taught by Diamond Way Ayurveda.

FIGURE 10–2 The six senses.

Western Medicine

Scientific progress throughout history developed into the more modern practices of Western medicine. Modern Western medicine takes a scientific approach to diagnosing the causes of health concerns and treating the symptoms (Figure 10–3). In recent times, the practice of Western medicine has lost many

FIGURE 10–3 Western medicine commonly entails counseling from a doctor.

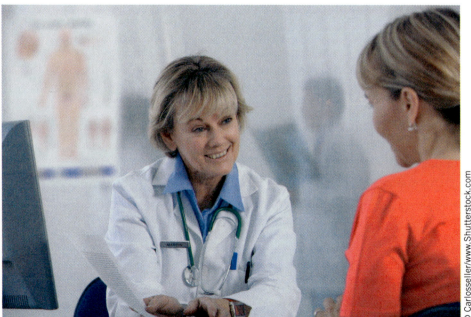

© Carlosseller/www.Shutterstock.com

of the characteristics it once shared with Eastern philosophy and has shifted to just dealing with symptoms. Currently, many Western physicians are moving to incorporate portions of both Eastern and Western approaches to treat the whole person, supporting scientific advances with alternative medicines to help the patient achieve the best health available.

Western medicine includes the following to evaluate the patient:

- Medical history
- Client feedback
- Physical examination based on symptoms
- Evaluation of the symptoms
- Blood and/or urine tests
- Diagnostic imaging, including X-rays, MRIs, and CAT scans
- Diagnostic surgery
- Other diagnostic tests based on symptoms

Western medicine incorporates the following to treat the patient:

- Oral and/or topical medications
- Injections
- Transfusions
- Chemotherapy
- Radiation
- Surgical techniques
- Physical therapy

Alternative Therapies

Alternative therapies add an Eastern philosophy dimension to Western medicine. Alternative therapies meld Eastern and the Western philosophies into a separate and distinctive category. Alternative therapies are becoming more commonly desired, as such a variety of possibilities is available.

Alternative therapies include the following treatment techniques:

- Hypnosis
- Biofeedback
- Reiki
- Acupuncture (Figure 10–4)
- Acupressure
- Stress management techniques
- Exercise techniques, including Pilates and yoga
- Nutritional counseling
- Weight management
- Herbal tinctures
- Floral essences
- Essential oil therapies
- Chiropractic therapies
- Osteopathic therapies
- Counseling

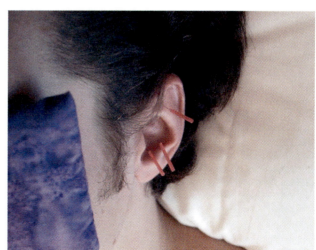

FIGURE 10–4 Acupuncture is a common form of alternative therapy.

© Cora Reed/www.Shutterstock.com

WELLNESS

Wellness is the promotion of habits that promote mental and physical soundness and lifelong health. Wellness is not restricted to the use of medications or medical care as it embraces a lifestyle of healthy eating, exercise, health care, and personal care. Wellness also includes a "feeling" of health that comes from the above characteristics plus internal mental balance. It is a balance of the physical, mental, and emotional or spiritual aspects of a person.

As estheticians, we are restricted in our scope of practice based on our licensure, which prohibits us from treating medical or mental disorders. These we should refer to licensed medical professionals. Nevertheless, we can provide a space that contributes to our own wellness and that of our client. Professional estheticians can set a positive example for clients by practicing wellness habits that will help our skin look its very best.

For personal wellness, we must practice:

- Healthy eating lifestyle
- Some form of exercise (compatible with our age, health, and physical ability) (Figure 10–5)
- Good work habits (grooming, professionalism, ethics)
- Personal growth time (education and learning)
- Personal reflection
- Personal renewal time (relaxation)

In a facility offering esthetic treatments, promotion of wellness can be more achievable in an ambiance that invites relaxation and calm and promotes wellness. Achieving such an atmosphere can be very simple or elaborate. Some sense-stimulating elements that you should consider for the treatment room include (Figure 10–6):

FIGURE 10–5 Pilates is a popular form of exercise.

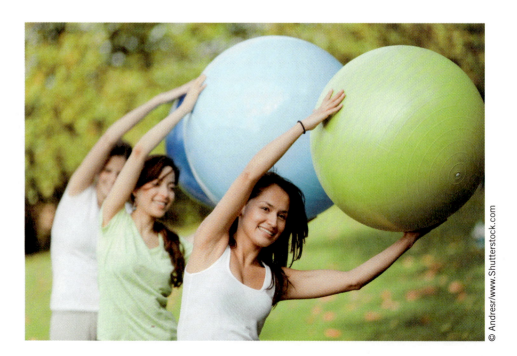

- Use of soothing colors
- Playing soothing, relaxing music
- Lighting style and effect
- Selections of fabric and textures in sheets, towels, robes
- Herbal teas
- Snacks of fruits and/or nuts
- Articles or brochures on healthy choices
- Articles or brochures on relaxation and stress reduction
- Alternative health services

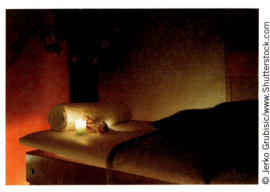

FIGURE 10–6 Example of ambiance that invites relaxation, calmness and promotes wellness.

© Jerko Grubisic/www.Shutterstock.com license from shutterstock.com.

Nutrition

Proper nutrition is vital to the health of an individual. When the body takes in nutrients, the vital internal organs and the brain are the first to be nourished. The last things to be fed are the skin, hair, and nails. Inadequate intake of nutrients can manifest as dry hair that may thin or not grow well; nails that split, peel, or are brittle; and skin that is dull, sallow-looking, and congested (with subsurface bumps). It is of utmost importance that proper nutrition be a priority in achieving a healthy body. Individualized proper nutrition can be achieved with self-education and planning (Figure 10–7). For more information, the Web site www.nutrition.gov offers a wide array of helpful articles. One major component of achieving proper nutrition includes using proper supplements if nutrients are not adequately provided in your diet. People must make informed food choices that include an understanding of food production and preparation. It is also important to consider the quality, quantity, and organization of daily food intake.

Water

Water is an essential nutrient that no human can live without. The body and skin depend on water to function properly. Drinking pure water offers the benefits of helping with sustaining cellular health, toxin and waste elimination, temperature regulation, and proper digestion. Water intake needs vary individually, but the average recommendation is to drink 9 to 12 cups of water each day.

Supplements

Supplements are dietary or nutritional additions to a daily diet (Figure 10–8). Some people may not consume adequate nutrients, vitamins, fiber, and fatty or amino acids. The FDA has set some minimum vitamin and mineral guidelines for daily consumption by children and adults. Ideally, everyone would get all of the nutrients necessary by consumption of foods in their most natural form. Natural forms of food items include those that are vine-ripened, unprocessed, and free of hormone additives in categories of fresh fruits, vegetables, proteins, and grains. Achieving this may be difficult due to local climates, dieting preferences, or lifestyles.

People also may have personal needs or strong personal food choices. Some people may prefer never to eat meat or starches, while others may consider both a necessity to the daily diet. Both groups may be missing nutrients and may benefit from supplements.

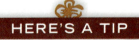

HERE'S A TIP

A self-assessment can determine whether supplements would be beneficial; in order to perform a self-assessment, carefully examine your skin, hair, and nails. Note the date on a calendar and begin supplements for 60 days. Then re-examine the condition of skin, hair, and nails. Check color, strength, and rate of growth.

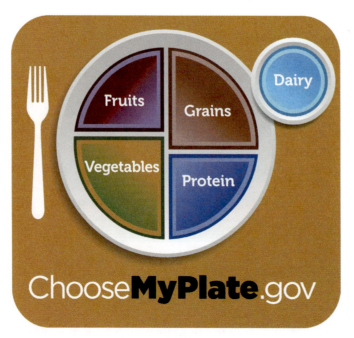

Vegetables	Fruits	Grains	Dairy	Protein Foods
Eat more red, orange, and dark-green veggies like tomatoes, sweet potatoes, and broccoli in main dishes. Add beans or peas to salads (kidney or chickpeas), soups (split peas or lentils), and side dishes (pinto or baked beans), or serve as a main dish. Fresh, frozen, and canned vegetables all count. Choose "reduced sodium" or "no-salt-added" canned veggies.	Use fruits as snacks, salads, and desserts. At breakfast, top your cereal with bananas or strawberries; add blueberries to pancakes. Buy fruits that are dried, frozen, and canned (in water or 100% juice), as well as fresh fruits. Select 100% fruit juice when choosing juices.	Substitute whole-grain choices for refined-grain breads, bagels, rolls, break-fast cereals, crackers, rice, and pasta. Check the ingredients list on product labels for the words "whole" or "whole grain" before the grain ingredient name. Choose products that name a whole grain first on the ingredients list.	Choose skim (fat-free) or 1% (low-fat) milk. They have the same amount of calcium and other essential nutrients as whole milk, but less fat and calories. Top fruit salads and baked potatoes with low-fat yogurt. If you are lactose intolerant, try lactose-free milk or fortified soymilk (soy beverage).	Eat a variety of foods from the protein food group each week, such as seafood, beans and peas, and nuts as well as lean meats, poultry, and eggs. Twice a week, make seafood the protein on your plate. Choose lean meats and ground beef that are at least 90% lean. Trim or drain fat from meat and remove skin from poultry to cut fat and calories.

For a 2,000-calorie daily food plan, you need the amounts below from each food group.
To find amounts personalized for you, go to Choose**MyPlate**.gov.

Eat 2½ cups every day	Eat 2 cups every day	Eat 6 ounces every day	Get 3 cups every day	Eat 5½ ounces every day
What counts as a cup? 1 cup of raw or cooked vegetables or vegetable juice; 2 cups of leafy salad greens	**What counts as a cup?** 1 cup of raw or cooked fruit or 100% fruit juice; ½ cup dried fruit	**What counts as an ounce?** 1 slice of bread; ½ cup of cooked rice, cereal, or pasta; 1 ounce of ready-to-eat cereal	**What counts as a cup?** 1 cup of milk, yogurt, or fortified soymilk; 1½ ounces natural or 2 ounces processed cheese	**What counts as an ounce?** 1 ounce of lean meat, poultry, or fish; 1 egg; 1 Tbsp peanut butter; ½ ounce nuts or seeds; ¼ cup beans or peas

U.S. Department of Agriculture • Center for Nutrition Policy and Promotion
August 2011
CNPP-25
USDA is an equal opportunity provider and employer.

FIGURE 10–7A,B The USDA *MyPlate*.

© Courtesy of U.S. Department of Agriculture.

It is suggested that each individual consider his or her average daily nutrition and seek out supplements for any necessary nutrients that may be lacking. More detailed information may be found at http://ods.od.nih.gov/, the site for the United States Office of Dietary Supplements. You should also discuss this with your personal physician or receive guidance from a nutritionist.

Not all supplements work equally well for all people. According to the United States Office of Dietary Supplements, before purchasing or using dietary supplements, you should keep a few things in mind:

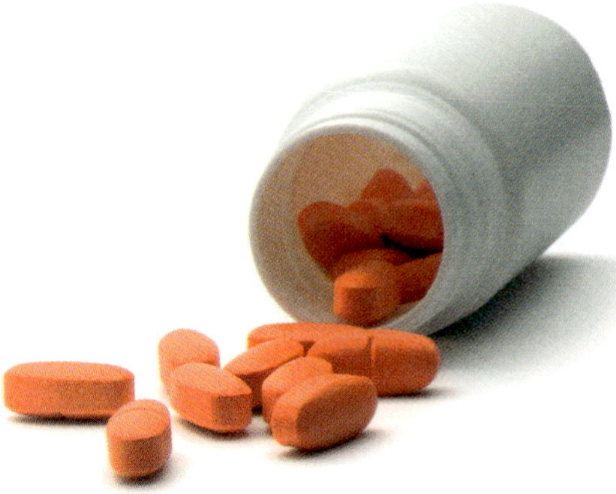

FIGURE 10-8 Supplements are dietary or nutritional additions to the daily diet.

© Trykster/www.Shutterstock.com

- Remember: Safety first. Some supplement ingredients, including nutrients and plant components, can be toxic based on their activity in your body. Do not substitute a dietary supplement for a prescription medicine or therapy.
- Think twice about chasing the latest headline. Sound health advice is generally based on research over time, not a single study touted by the media. Be wary of results claiming a "quick fix" that depart from scientific research and established dietary guidance.
- Learn to spot false claims. Remember: "If something sounds too good to be true, it probably is." Some examples of false claims on product labels:
  ○ Quick and effective "cure-all."
  ○ Can treat or cure disease.
  ○ "Totally safe," "all-natural," and has "definitely no side effects."
  ○ Limited availability, "no-risk, money-back guarantee," or requires advance payment.
- More may not be better. Some products can be harmful when consumed in high amounts, for a long time, or in combination with certain other substances.
- The term "natural" doesn't always mean safe. Do not assume that this term ensures wholesomeness or safety. For some supplements, "natural" ingredients may interact with medicines, be dangerous for people with certain health conditions, or be harmful in high doses. For example, tea made from peppermint leaves is generally considered safe to drink, but peppermint oil (extracted from the leaves) is much more concentrated and can be toxic if used incorrectly.
- Is the product worth the money? Resist the pressure to buy a product or treatment "on the spot." Some supplement products may be expensive or may not provide the benefit you expect. For example, excessive amounts of water-soluble vitamins, like vitamin C and B vitamins, are not used by the body and are eliminated in the urine.

When selecting supplements, it is also recommended to seek those that are "standardized" to be assured that they contain what they claim. The United States Pharmacopeia (USP) tests supplements to determine their quality and ability to be dissolved. Looking for USP verification on a product label is a good way to be sure that the supplement you are purchasing will properly offer benefits.

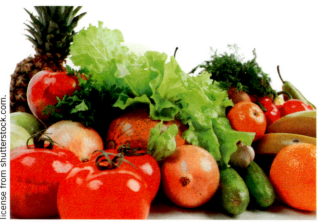

FIGURE 10–9 The term "organic" refers to the way agricultural products are grown and processed.

Organics

The word "organic" refers to the way farmers grow and process agricultural products such as fruits, vegetables, grains, dairy products, and meat (Figure 10–9). Organic farming may offer economic and environmental benefits. Some consumers have sensitivities to products used in the conventional farming process that may be eliminated by consuming organically produced food items.

Educating yourself about the benefits of organics and what food products qualify as organic can be beneficial to your nutritional choices. A good place to begin is by checking labels and looking for the United States Department of Agriculture (USDA) organic label. Standards have been developed by the USDA that regulates how foods are grown, handled, and processed.

You may see other terms on food labels, such as "all-natural," "free-range" or "hormone-free." These descriptions may be important to you, but don't confuse them with the term "organic." Only those foods that are grown and processed according to USDA organic standards can be labeled organic. Educate yourself on reading food labels so you can make informed choices for maximum benefits.

Inadequate Nutrition

Many factors may affect whether we get adequate nutrition. Inadequate amounts of nutrients available to the body may be a result of:

- Diets heavily dependent on fast foods (high in fats and grease)
- Cutting out foods to control weight
- Diets low in fruits and vegetables
- Unavailability of vine-ripened fruits or vegetables
- Inadequate amounts of protein
- Diets high in refined sugars or processed foods
- High caffeine intake
- Medications that compromise nutrient absorption
- Gastrointestinal disorders that compromise nutrient absorption
- High alcohol intake
- Inadequate rest
- High stress levels

FYI

Vitamin and herbal supplements may cause a conflict with other drug treatments. Always advise clients to give their healthcare provider complete information concerning all the substances they consume.

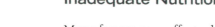

Did You Know?

Organic food products purchased from local growers will not always carry the USDA seal verifying that they were grown organically. This is because smaller agriculture producers are not required to be registered as organic growers through the USDA. They are still expected to follow the same guidelines if labeling their items organic.

Good nutrition is about making food choices that will provide the nutrients that body needs in adequate amounts (Figure 10–10). Poor food choices can actually lead to more hunger as the body tries to get what it is missing. Excess fats, sugars, and starches are stored, leading to weight gain. The extra weight can lead to other health issues or crash dieting. Adequate nutrition provides the body with the vitamins it needs to maintain good health. Adequate vitamin intake also has many esthetic benefits. Lack of sufficient vitamins in the diet can stress the body. The body may suffer from lack of nutrition for any number of reasons; two specific ones to be aware of are glycation and crash dieting.

Glycation

Glycation is a destructive process that leads to the cross-linking of body fibers and accelerated aging. External glycation of food items is caused during the cooking process, when sugars and starch react with proteins under high temperature. Internal glycation is associated with increased oxidative damage. The result of both types of glycation is the formation of advanced glycation end products (AGEs). AGEs are known contributors for numerous diseases including the following:

- Alzheimer's disease
- Cataract formation
- Type II diabetes
- Heart disease
- Obesity
- Premature aging of the skin

This process commonly occurs when foods are fried, seared, barbequed, broiled, grilled, or baked at high temperatures (Figure 10–11). All of these result in "browning" of the food, which enhances its flavor and makes it more desirable. The resulting flavors are used in the food flavoring industry; glycated proteins may be present in your food even if the final preparation is not done at a high temperature. While we may not be able to eliminate glycation, we can reduce it by cooking at low temperatures. Low-temperature preparation techniques such as slow cooking, stewing, and poaching are preferred.

Many naturally low-AGE-content food items are available for consumption; some are listed here (Figure 10–12):

- Dairy products—low-fat
- Fruit—small quantities and minimize dried fruits

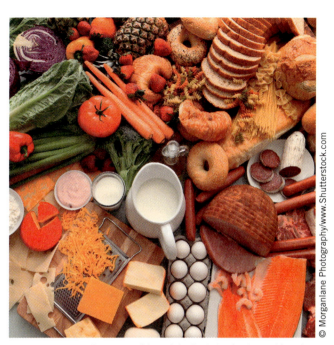

FIGURE 10–10 Proper nutrition of the body begins by making the right choices.

© Morganlane Photography/www.Shutterstock.com

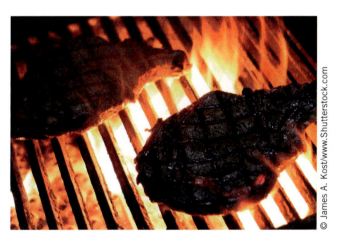

FIGURE 10–11 Barbecued foods contain high levels of AGE products.

© James A. Kost/www.Shutterstock.com

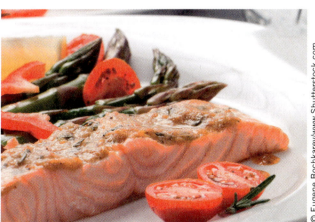

FIGURE 10–12 Many food items have low AGE content.

© Eugene Bochkarev/www.Shutterstock.com

- Grains
- Legumes
- Nuts
- Vegetables
- Fish—not fried or breaded

Crash Dieting

"Crash dieting" is a term that describes extreme cutbacks in food quantity in an effort to lose weight. These cutbacks are often achieved by counting calories consumed and taking in far less than is needed for body maintenance, which is a form of starvation dieting. Other forms of crash dieting may include the elimination of one or more food groups. Any form of crash dieting commonly occurs in conjunction with extreme exercise routines or use of diet pills.

Some examples of crash or "fad" diets include:

- Liquid diets
- Cabbage soup diet
- Grapefruit diet
- Bananas and milk diet
- Maple syrup diet
- Low-calorie diets
- Low-carbohydrate diets
- Anti-cellulite diets

CAUTION

People have suffered serious health consequences and even death from crash dieting. Such diets are considered extremely dangerous by medical professionals and dieticians.

The goal of the extreme cutbacks is to get the body to use its stored fat. With this method, the body is not receiving a balance of nutrients and so it may begin to metabolize muscle tissue instead of fat to get the components it needs to sustain life. While the dieter may initially lose some weight, this is water weight loss. After a period of time, the person will plateau and find it difficult to lose any more weight. The body adjusts its metabolism so that it can get by on fewer calories, so as soon as the person goes off the diet, the body will regain weight even faster than before. Crash dieting is tied into yo-yo dieting, where the person gets trapped in a cycle of weight gain and loss, each time regaining the weight more easily and quickly. Exacerbating the cycle, the person often returns to the pre-diet food choices that caused the weight gain in the first place.

During the diet, the person's general health and the skin, hair, and nails all suffer due to inadequate levels of nutrients being consumed. Estheticians cannot give nutritional counseling, but we should encourage good, healthy eating. Fad diets do not provide adequate nutrients and should be discouraged. If a client is determined to try a fad diet for a short period of time, encourage him or her to seek the advice of a nutritionist and take proper supplements. Crash dieting has numerous detrimental side effects, including vitamin deficiencies and mood swings.

FYI

Even though you may be sincerely concerned about your clients' health, avoid the temptation to give specific advice about vitamin or herbal supplements.

Lifestyle Diets

Numerous lifestyle diets are available and can be safely recommended. These types of nationally recognized diets are concerned with healthy eating lifestyles. The diets work to educate people in making food choices that will result in better long-term health and weight management. A person who wishes to lose weight will exercise portion control, but never to the extent of crash dieting. Instead, the weight loss will be slower as the person is retrained in a new eating lifestyle. Food choices and portion control are stressed as lifelong habits. When a healthy weight is achieved, food portions are adjusted to assure long-term adequate intake of nutrients without weight rebound. Dietary supplements are often recommended to assure proper levels of nutrients are maintained. Safe lifestyle diet recommendations include:

- American Heart Association diet
- American Diabetes Association diet
- American Cancer Association diet

For other popular diets like Weight Watchers, the Zone diet, the South Beach diet, or the Atkins diet, consider referring your client to their physician to see if they are suitable for them. Descriptions of diet programs may be found at www .WebMD.com, along with medical reviews and pros and cons for each program.

Any of the above diets could be adapted to specific food-choice lifestyles such as vegetarianism or veganism. Those following vegetarian and vegan lifestyles must be make a special effort to obtain adequate protein from their diets.

All diets should be accompanied by some form of exercise. In addition to burning off calories, exercise stimulates the body's metabolism and circulation and the proper functioning of the digestive system.

Stress Management

The human body becomes stressed when a "trigger" stimulates a hormonal response. The trigger may be an event, encounter, or other incident. The automatic stress response dates back to our ancient ancestors, who had to decide in a moment how to respond to a potentially threatening situation. Often referred to as the fight-or-flight response, the decision hinged on whether our ancestors believed that they could fight off a potential attacker or that flight—escape—was the better alternative.

This is an instinctive and natural human response. When a cause of stress is presented, a cascade of chemical events occurs in the brain and the adrenal glands secrete a hormonal response. The senses become more alert and our bodies shift into quick-response mode. This allows us to achieve things we might not be able to under normal circumstances. The chain of response includes the following reactions:

- Release of adrenaline
- Release of cortisol
- Heart rate increases
- Muscles tighten
- Blood pressure rises
- Breathing quickens
- Senses sharpen
- Strength, stamina, reaction time, and focus accelerate

The surge of hormones only lasts a short time, just long enough to allow us to respond and escape from danger. Then the body will begin to regroup and attempt to work toward the pre-stress state. If we were trying to escape from heavy traffic, we might be tempted to hit the accelerator to drive faster but keep our other foot hovering over the brake in case we needed to stop abruptly. Unfortunately, in today's world this speed–brake dilemma often repeats itself over and over again. Busy lifestyles may cause frequent progression from one stressor to another without offering the body a reprieve.

Some common causes of increased or sudden stress include:

- Loss of a loved one
- Changes in family status
- Relationship issues
- Changes in work status
- Personal injury or illness
- Changes in schedule, routine, or activities
- Moving
- Changes in sleep patterns or habits
- Fears and anxiety
- Perfectionism or cynicism
- Financial situations
- Social situations
- Holidays
- Vacations
- Changes in responsibilities at home or work
- Changes in arguments (pattern, frequency, intensity)
- Pregnancy
- Small spaces
- Hot rooms
- Loud music
- Unbalanced diet

Chronic stress is stress that has become habitual and ongoing, without an end to it in sight. Dealing with work, children, finances, and other obligations is part of chronic stress. The energy created by the stressor is not used up and the buildup of adrenaline and cortisol in the body begins to wear on the natural defense system.

Common symptoms of chronic stress include:

- Headaches (Figure 10–13)
- Fatigue
- Interrupted sleep patterns
- Weight gain
- Anxiety
- Memory issues
- Difficulty concentrating
- Increased mistakes
- Depression
- Weakened immune system
- Skin irritations or hives
- Loss of nutrient reserves

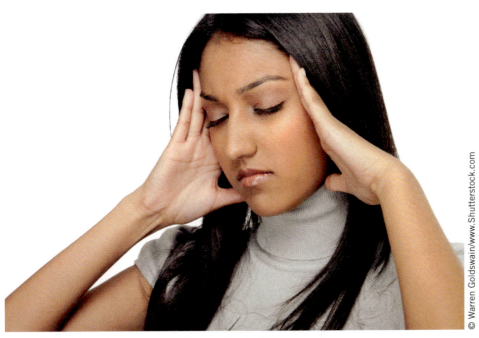

FIGURE 10–13 Headaches are a symptom of chronic stress.

It is important to identify stress triggers that affect us and recognize that what stresses one person may not affect another in the same way. Some people use food when they get stressed, but this can lead to other issues such as weight gain. As estheticians, we can offer suggestions to our clients on dealing with stress in non-food ways such as:

- Deep controlled breathing
- Deliberately slowing speech and movements
- Deliberately calming down
- Going for a walk (Figure 10–14)
- Allowing yourself to make choices about what you will and will not do
- Meditation
- Exercise
- Relaxation

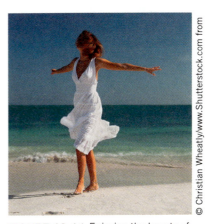

FIGURE 10–14 Enjoying the beauty of nature has a calming effect.

FINDING BALANCE

In the hectic lifestyles found in our society, it is important for the esthetician to seek personal balance (Figure 10–15). This means finding a balance between the demands of career, family, and personal needs. If we can work toward finding this balance for ourselves, it will be easier to help our clients find it also. Many estheticians are self-employed, which means they face the demands not just of providing quality services and customer care but dealing with all aspects of running a business. If they are trying to do this in addition to meeting the needs of a growing family, the stress level can become overwhelming and lead to negative results.

Traditionally, society has taught women from childhood to take care of others while men are seen as being financially responsible for the household. For many

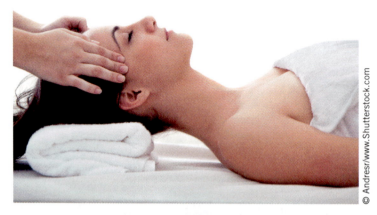

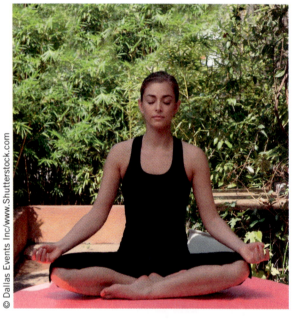

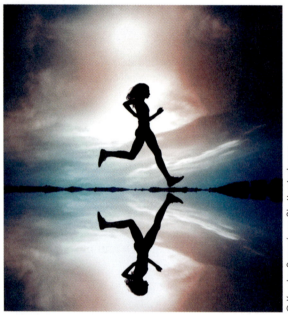

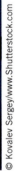

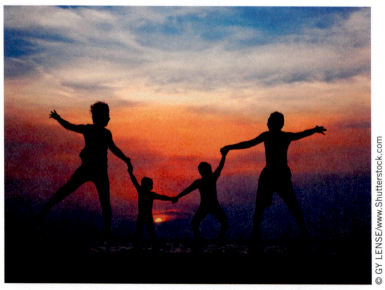

FIGURE 10–15A,B,C,D Balance is achieved through a variety of methods including relaxation, meditation, exercise, and quality time with family.

women, this means putting others' needs above any caring for self, which can lead to chronic stress. Men may feel pressure to achieve a certain status or success level. Schedules or time management practices offer dedication to priorities such as to home and family and the workplace. Personal care, rest, relaxation, and fun are equally important to a healthy lifestyle.

General Wellness Plan

A plan of general wellness includes the following:

- Diet
  - Eat a variety of foods for balance and limit or omit unhealthy items.
  - Take daily supplements.
  - Drink adequate amounts of water.
- Exercise
  - Make an effort to practice aerobic exercise three or more times a week for 20 to 30 minutes each.
  - Practice exercises to build core muscle strength and balance.
  - Warm up and cool down with each exercise session.
  - Stretch daily.
- Rest
  - Receive adequate sleep; six to nine hours are recommended.
  - Take short breaks during the day.
  - Enjoy a relaxing day on a weekly basis.
  - Take time for vacation at least once a year.
- Spirit
  - Meditate daily to help center yourself.
  - Know your sense of purpose in life and help others find theirs.
  - Enjoy and reflect on nature.
  - If you have religious beliefs, practice these often.
- Fun and Recreation
  - Find hobbies you enjoy that allow you to express yourself creatively.
  - Experience recreational hobbies such as dance, hiking, or gardening.
  - Look for social groups with shared interests, such as sports, reading clubs or, community service organizations.

Finding balance within yourself will allow you to feel better and enjoy life, and will lead to a more successful esthetic career. Educate yourself to find the most beneficial forms of health care, diet, exercise, and lifestyle for your individual needs. Be an example of leading a balanced lifestyle. The benefits of achieving health and wellness are clearly visible to others and will serve as motivation to clients, family, and coworkers.

Medical Information

HIPAA FOR ESTHETICIANS

The Health Insurance Portability and Accountability Act (HIPAA) of 1996 became effective on April 14, 2003; the intent of this regulation is to protect patient privacy regarding medical records and health information provided to health plans, doctors, hospitals, and other health care providers. The U.S. Department of Health and Human Services (HHS) developed this standard to provide patients with access to their medical records and help them gain greater control over how their personal health information is used.

The ease with which advancing technology can transfer private information has made some people reluctant to share critical information with their physicians or other health care providers, including pharmacists. HIPAA was created to give the public confidence and encourage full disclosure of medical concerns without worry of privacy intrusions. All employees are required to complete HIPAA training and have an understanding of and follow HIPAA rules. A complete description of the standard is available at www.hhs.gov/works

CONTROL OF CLIENT INFORMATION

Controlling client information is the key to safeguarding client privacy. Because estheticians collect sensitive medical information about clients, they must observe the strictly enforced requirements of the HIPAA laws. Here are the key standards of patient protection:

- **Access to medical records:** patients are able to see and receive copies of their medical records (this may also apply to esthetic records).
- **Notice of privacy practices:** health care providers must provide a notice to their patients on how they may use their personal medical information.
- **Limits use of personal medical information:** HIPAA stipulates that health care providers can only share patient information on a *need-to-know* basis.
- **Prohibits the use of patient information for marketing:** permission must be obtained from the patient to use personal medical information for other purposes.
- **Stronger state laws:** all states must comply with privacy standards.
- **Confidential communications:** patients can request that health care providers ensure that all communications are kept confidential.
- **Complaints:** patients can file formal complaints regarding a breach of confidentiality.

Keeping accurate records that comply with HIPAA standards is crucial in order to protect client confidentiality and ensure quality of care. One of the best techniques for this is to use proper documentation and storage of the documentation. Computerized information banks should be encrypted and password-protected.

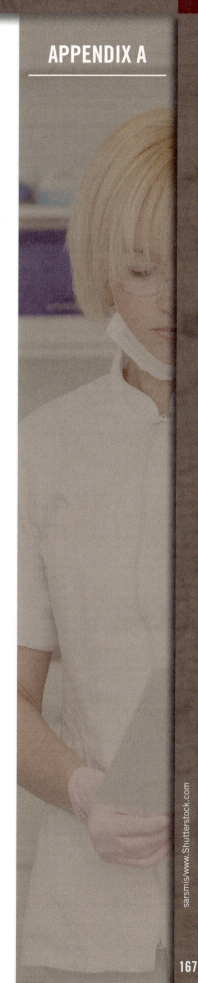

SOAP NOTES

SOAP notes are a popular method of documenting the critical thinking process. They are mandated in medical settings and have been adopted by many estheticians. SOAP notes ensure consistency, confidentiality, and thorough, effective analysis and communication. SOAP is an acronym for the four steps that should be followed during every client interaction.

- **S – Subjective:** what the client tells you
- **O – Objective:** what you see
- **A – Assessment:** details of what you observe
- **P – Procedure:** steps to take for the desired outcome

"Subjective" refers to information from the client's perspective. The technician should documented what treatments the client is requesting, a visual description of the client, and what the client desires to accomplish. "Objective" is the technician's initial observations of the client and a review of the subjective information provided. "Assessment" refers to the technician's findings when performing a detailed skin analysis under a magnifying lamp. The assessment also points to any correlation between what the client's goals are and what results are achievable. The "procedure" portion will include home care that the client will need to follow to meet esthetic goals, current treatment protocols, and the treatment series plan that will help the client achieve long-term goals.

CLIENT SAFETY AND HIPAA

Only rarely in an esthetics practice do situations involve domestic violence or other risks to the client. A situation in which an esthetician, massage therapist, or other health care provider suspects that a client is at risk is the only time that the need for intervention overrides client privacy issues.

Included in the duty to warn codes are potential child abuse, spousal abuse, and elder abuse. These are very delicate situations, so having the proper authorities to refer to is crucial to proper handling. Begin with your local law enforcement office when looking for the appropriate contact agency.

Abuse occurs in many ways. Some signs to be aware of include the following:

- Bruises
- Swelling
- Hematomas

REGULATION ALERT

Some states require not only health care providers but also other therapists to report to the authorities any clients who have intent to hurt others or hurt themselves. Each state has an official regulation and law Web site that provides state-specific details on law mandates for intent to harm. Technicians who do not comply may be breaking the law.

- Burns
- Bite marks
- Fractures
- Flinching when touched
- Poor hygiene
- Withdrawn posture
- Inability or unwillingness to make eye contact
- Poor nutritional states

INCIDENT DOCUMENTATION

Any first-aid treatments should be documented, and a written record of the events should follow standardized protocol. Include in the documentation the events leading up to the injury, the type of injury, and the steps taken to care for the person. Documentation should include the facts discovered following the incident. Include date and times of first-aid treatments and any change in the person's condition.

In the event that the incident requiring first-aid treatments involves an exposure to toxic or corrosive materials, include a copy of the Material Safety Data Sheet (MSDS). Provide a copy of the first-aid treatment record to the individual or EMS so the treating medical personnel have access to the incident documentation.

Pointers for incident documentation include the following:

- Be neat, thorough, and accurate.
- Record facts, NOT opinions.
- Describe the incident, including persons involved or witnesses.
- Describe any injury.
- Describe any steps taken following the incident, including any first aid administered.
- Sign, date, and keep a copy of your report.
- Complete the form as soon after the incident as possible. The longer the time frame, the more likely critical information will be missed.

When providing care for a victim of an accident or other incident, anything that is learned in the course of providing care is considered confidential. Do not share this information with anyone except EMS personnel directly associated with the client's medical care. Sharing personal information may constitute a breach of the client's privacy rights.

MEDICATIONS AND THE IMPACT ON SKIN

Many clients take a variety of herbs, supplements, and prescription medications. Knowledge of what they are taking and how the products can impact the skin will help the esthetician better select treatments appropriate for the specific client. Each of the following tables includes the category of drugs, examples of drugs in each category, and common skin effects that must be considered. Drugs are divided into categories based on the condition or disease that the drugs target. According to the FDA, there are over 35 drug categories. The following tables deal with some of the most common drugs that clients take.

Topical Medications

Topical medications may be either over-the-counter or prescription drugs.

Oral Medications

The following tables are divided by the purpose for which the oral medication is taken. These tables list the drug category, examples of the drugs, and common effects of the drug on the skin.

CATEGORY OF DRUG	EXAMPLES	COMMON SKIN EFFECTS
Anti-aging product	glycolic, lactic, retinols	redness, flakiness
Anti-acne	benzoyl-peroxide, salicylic	redness, flakiness

TABLE 1 Common Over-the-Counter Topical Drugs

CATEGORY OF DRUG	EXAMPLES	COMMON SKIN EFFECTS
Anti-aging	Retin-A, Renova	redness, flakiness, irritation, itching, scaling, burning
Antibiotics	Cleocin-T, ClinaDerm	burning, itching, dryness, redness
Antivirals	Denavir, Zovirax	headaches, redness, burning, stinging
Anti-inflammatory	Aclovate	stinging, itching, redness, infection, thinning of skin

TABLE 2 Common Prescription Topical Drugs

DRUG CATEGORY	EXAMPLE	COMMON SKIN EFFECTS
Hormones	Calcitonin, Danazol, Desmopressin, Epoetin, estrogens, Estropipate, Fludrocortisone, Glucagon, insulins, Leuprolide, Levothyroxine, Liothyronine, Liotrix, Megestrol, Nafarelin, Nandrolone decanoate, progestins, Teriparatide, vasopressin	rashes, acne, hirsutism, oily skin, itching, flushing, hyperpigmentation, hives
Birth control medications	estradiol acetate, estradiol cypionate, estradiol cypionate, estradiol valerate, estradiol topical emulsion, estradiol transdermal system, estradiol vaginal tablet, estradiol vaginal ring, ethinyl estradiol/desogestrel, ethinyl estradiol/drospirenone, ethinyl estradiol/ethynodiol, ethinyl estradiol/etonogestrel, ethinyl estradiol/levonorgestrel, ethinyl estradiol/norelgestromin, ethinyl estradiol/norethindrone, ethinyl estradiol/norgestimate, ethinyl estradiol/norgestrel, levonorgestrel, levonorgestrel/ethinyl estrodiol, medroxyprogesterone, mestranol/norethindrone, norethindrone, norethindrone/ethinyl acetate, norgestimate/ethinyl estradiol, Norgestrel	acne, hirsutism, oily skin, rashes, itching, flushing, hyperpigmentation, hives

TABLE 3 Hormones

DRUG CATEGORY	EXAMPLE	COMMON SKIN EFFECTS
Lipid-lowering agents	Choletyramine, colesevlam, colestipol, atorvastatin, fluvastatin, lovastatin, pravastatin, rosuvastatin, simvastatin	Irritation, rashes
Antithrombolytics	Argatroban, bivalirudin, desirudin, lepirudin, anistreplase, streptokinase, tenecteplase	Ecchymoses, flushing, hives
Anticoagulants	Heparin and warfarin	Alopecia, rashes, hives, dermal necrosis
Antiplatelets	Dalteparin, enoxaparin, fondaparinux, tinzaparin, eptifibatide, tirofiban	Ecchymoses, itching, rash, hives, bruising

TABLE 4 Drugs That Affect the Blood

DRUG CATEGORY	EXAMPLE	COMMON SKIN EFFECTS
Beta blockers	Atenolol, carteolol, labetalol, metoprolol, nadolol, propranolol	Dermatitis, **erythema multiforme**, flushing, increased sweating, itching, rashes
Calcium channel blockers	Diltiazem, felodipine, isradipine, nicardipine, verapamil	Dermatitis, erythema multiforme, flushing, increased sweating, hives
Nitrates	Isosorbide mononitrate, isosorbide dinitrate, nitroglycerin	Skin rash, yellowing of the skin, contact dermatitis, flushing of face and neck, bluish-colored lips, fingernails, or palms of hands
Antiarrhythmics	Disopyramide, moricizine, procainamide, quinidine, fosphenytoin, mexiletine, tocainide, acebutolol, diltiazem, atropine	Itching, skin rash, yellowing of the skin, dermatitis, erythema multiforme, flushing, increased sweating, **photosensitivity**, pruritus/urticaria
Antihypertensives	Clonidine, eplerenone, benazepril, captopril, lisinopril, moexipril, ramipril, guanfacine methyldopa, doxazosin, candesartan	Flushing, rash, itching, hives, sweating

TABLE 5 Common Drugs Used to Treat Heart Conditions

DRUG CATEGORY	EXAMPLE	COMMON SKIN EFFECTS
Antihistamines	Azatadine, clemastine, bromopheniramine, diphenhydramine, fexofenadine, loratadine, epinephrine	Erythema, photosensitivity, excessive sweating, rash, and hives
Antiasthmatics	Cromolyn, nedocromil, zafirlukast, albuterol, formoterol, levalbuterol, salmeterol, montelukast	Rash, erythema, flushing, hives, photosensitivity
Bronchodilators	Formoterol, levalbuterol, terbutiline, theophylline	Rash, erythema, flushing, hives, photosensitivity

TABLE 6 Common Drugs Used to Treat Lung Disorders

DRUG CATEGORY	EXAMPLE	COMMON SKIN EFFECTS
Anticholinergics	Atropine, darifenacin, dicyclomine, hyoscyamine, oxybutynin, solifenacin, tolteradine	Urticaria, flushing and decreased sweating
Antidiarrheals	Bismuth subsalicylate, difenoxin/atropine, diphenoxylate, kaolin/pectin, loperamide	Flushing
Antiemetics	Dolasetron, ondansetron, granisetron	Pruritis
Antiulcer drugs	Aluminum hydroxide, magnesium hydroxide/aluminum hydroxide, esomeprazole, lansoprazole, omeprazole, rabeprazole, cimetidine, famotidine, nizatidine, randitine, sodium bicarbonate, calcium acetate, magnesium hydroxide	Pruritis, flushing, sweating, photosensitivity and rash

TABLE 7 Common Drugs Used to Treat Gastrointestinal Disorders

DRUG CATEGORY	EXAMPLE	COMMON SKIN EFFECTS
Antianxiety drugs	Alprazolam, chlordiazepoxide, diazepam, lorazepam, midazolam, oxazpam	Rashes
Anticonvulsants	Buspirone, doxepin, hydroxyzine pamoate, hydroxyzine hydrochloride, paroxetine hydrochloride, venlafaxine, phenobarbital, phenytoin, divalproex sodium, valproate sodium, valproic acid	Rashes, hypertrichosis, exfoliative dermatitis, pruritis, ecchymoses, photosensitivity, rashes, flushing
Antidepressants	Citalopram, duloxetine hydrochloride, escitalopram, fluoxetine, paroxetine, sertraline, mirtazapine, nortriptyline, phenelzine, trazodone, bupropion	Ecchymoses, pruritis, photosensitivity, rashes, itching, hives, alopecias
Antipsychotics	Clozapine, olanzapine, haloperidol, quetiapine, risperidone, ziprasidone	Rash, hives and sweating, dry skin, sun sensitivity, ecchymoses, pruritis
Central nervous system stimulants	Amphetamine mixtures, dextroamphetamine, methylphenidate	Unusual bruising, hives, rash and itching
Sedatives	Chloral hydrate, droperidol, eszopiclone, ramelteon, zaleplon, zolpidem	Rashes, photosensitivity, sweating

TABLE 8 Common Drugs Used to Treat Mental Disorders

DRUG CATEGORY	EXAMPLE	COMMON SKIN EFFECTS
Antibiotics	Amikacin, kanamycin, neomycin, streptomycin, tobramycin, ertapenem, meropenem, cefadroxil monohydrate, cefazolin, cephalexin, cefotetan, cefuroxime, loracarbef, cefoperazone, ceftriaxone, piperacillin, ticarcillin, ciprofloxacin, levofloxacin, moxfloxacin, norfloxacin, ofloxacin, azithromycin clarithromycin, erythromycin, amoxicillin, ampicillin, cloxacillin, dicloxacillin, oxacillin, nafcillin, penicillin, doxycycline, minocycline, tetracycline, clindamycin, metronidazole, vancomycin	Rashes, itching, burning, photosensitivity, rashes and hives with topical use, mild dryness, skin irritation, transient redness, epidermal necrolysis, erythema multiforme

TABLE 9 Common Antibiotics

DRUG CATEGORY	EXAMPLE	COMMON SKIN EFFECTS
Antivirals	Acyclovir, amantadine hydrochloride, cidofovir, docosanol, entecavir, famciclovir, ganciclovir, lamivudine, oseltamivir, penciclovir, ribavrin, valacyclovir, valganciclovir hydrochloride, vidarabine, zanamivir, delavirdine mesylate, efavirenz, nevirapine, abacavir, didanosine, emtriciabine, stavudine, zalcitabine, zidovudine	Acne, hives, rashes, sweating, Stevens Johnson syndrome, hair loss, dry, itchy skin, photosensitivity, erythema multiforme, hives, ecchymoses, nail pigmentation, lipodystrophy

TABLE 10 Common Drugs Used to Treat Viruses

DRUG CATEGORY	EXAMPLE	COMMON SKIN EFFECTS
Systemic antifungals	Amphotericin B, fluconazole, itraconazole, terbinafine, voriconazole	Flushing, exfoliative skin disorders, Stevens Johnson syndrome, rash, itching, toxic epidermal necrolysis, and photosensitivity
Topical antifungals	Butenafine, butoconazole, ciclopirox, clotrimazole, econazole, haloprogin, ketoconazole, miconazole, nystatin, oxiconazole, sulconazole, tolnaftate	Burning, itching, local sensitivity, redness, stinging, local irritation, sensitization, rash or itching, hives, toxic epidermal necrolysis

TABLE 11 Common Drugs Used to Treat Fungal Infections

DRUG CATEGORY	EXAMPLE	COMMON SKIN EFFECTS
Osteoporosis drugs	Alendronate, Etidronate, Pamidronate risedronate, Tiludronate, Zoledronic acid, Raloxifene	Itching, swelling, skin rash, sweating, flushing, photosensitivity, erythema multiforme
Rheumatoid arthritis drugs	Anakinra, Etanercept, Hydroxychloroquine, Infliximab, Leflunomide, Methotrexate, Cyclosporine, Sulfasalazine	Rashes, exfoliative dermatitis, photosensitivity, yellow discoloration of the skin, hirsutism, acne, hives and skin ulcers, alopecia, painful plaque erosions, photosensitivity

TABLE 12 Common Drugs Used to Treat Skeletal Conditions

DRUG CATEGORY	EXAMPLE	COMMON SKIN EFFECTS
Corticosteroids	Beclomethasone, budesonide, flunisolide, fluticasone, triamcinolone, beclomethasone, budesonide, fluticasone, mometasone, loteprednol, prednisolone, rimexolone, hydrocortisone, cortisone, prednisolone, prednisone, dexamethasone, alclometasone, clocortolone, desoximetasone, diflorasone, flucinonide	Acne, delayed wound healing, ecchymoses, fragile skin integrity, hirsutism, petechiae, allergic contact dermatitis, skin shrinking, burning, dryness, swelling, folliculitis, hypersensitivity, hypertrichoses, loss of pigmentation, irritation, maceration, miliaria, perioral dermatitis, secondary infections, stretch marks

TABLE 13 Corticosteroids

DRUG CATEGORY	EXAMPLE	COMMON SKIN EFFECTS
Narcotic analgesics	Buprenorphine, butorphanol, codeine, fentanyl citrate, fentanyl transdermal system, hydrocodone, hydromorphone, meperidine hydrochloride, methadone, morphine, nalbuphine, oxycodone, oxymorphone, propoxyphene	Pruritus, rash, flushing, urticaria, exfoliative dermatitis
Non-steroidal anti-inflammatory agents (NSAIDs)	Celecoxib, diclofenac, diflunisal, etodolac, fenoprofen, flurbiprofen, ibuprofen, indomethacin, ketoprofen, ketorolac, meloxicam, nabumetone, naproxen, oxaprozin, piroxicam, sulindac, tolmetin	Stevens Johnson syndrome and exfoliative dermatitis, ecchymoses, skin rash, and itching
Non-narcotic analgesics	Acetaminophen, butalbital compounds, capsaicin, choline and magnesium, salicylates, salsalate	Dermatitis, rash, exfoliative dermatitis, Stevens Johnson syndrome, toxic epidermal necrolysis
Muscle relaxants	Baclofen, carisoprodol, chlorzoxazone, cyclobenzaprine, dantrolene, diazepam, metaxalone, methocarbamol, orphenadrine	Flushing, pruritis, rash, urticaria, sweating

TABLE 14 Common Drugs Used to Treat Pain

HERBS AND SUPPLEMENTS

Most supplements and herbs do not generally pose health risks, but do pose a risk when taken in large doses or when combined with other medications. For estheticians, the most common concerns are remedies or supplements that may thin the blood, leaving the client more prone to bruising. This is not generally an issue for a normal, healthy person, and only becomes a concern if a client is consuming large quantities of some herbal remedies and is also on a prescription blood thinner. Foods that we eat seem to be balanced between those that may have a blood-thinning action and those that promote coagulation. Always encourage clients to discuss taking any herbal remedy or supplement with a medical professional.

Herbs and supplements that contribute to blood thinning include:

- Gingko biloba
- Ginger
- Garlic
- Dong quai
- Feverfew
- St. John's wort
- Coenzyme Q10
- Omega-3 fatty acids
- Cinnamon
- Vitamin E

Herbs and supplements that can promote clotting include:

- Ginseng
- Vitamin K
- Arnica montana

ESSENTIAL OIL CONSIDERATIONS

Because essential oils are highly concentrated substances, estheticians must receive training on the use of essential oils before incorporating them into their practice. Some essential oils may cause negative results in some clients, including allergic reactions, irritation, or reactions with existing health concerns. Always begin essential oil use with a manufacturer's preblended formula and expand as knowledge and experience progress.

Safety tips for incorporating essential oils:

- Check client history for potential contraindications and allergies.
- Always dilute essential oils before applying to the skin.
- Due to the link between smell and memory, allow the client to sniff the oil to make sure it is pleasant to them.

Protecting patient privacy must be ranked as a high priority by every esthetician. Knowing when and how to document incidents will offer peace of mind and protection in unfortunate situations. Complete a thorough intake form for every client and update the form on subsequent visits. Be familiar with potential side effects of all drugs.

FYI

Many clients do not consider herbal remedies to be medications and are often unaware that there may be potential drug interactions. Always encourage clients to discuss taking any supplement with a medical professional.

Safety- and Esthetics-Related Contacts

SAFETY-RELATED CONTACTS

It is important to have a complete list of safety-related contacts. This list should be reviewed and updated regularly in case there are changes. Check your local phone book or the Internet and develop your personalized, quick-to-use reference list. Look up the numbers and fill in the blanks for a quick referral guide.

Safety-Related Web Sites

Medline Plus	www.nlm.nih.gov/medlineplus/
National Institutes of Health	www.nih.gov
NOAA National Weather Service	www.weather.gov
NOAA Storm Prediction Center	www.spc.noaa.gov
Ready.gov (emergency preparedness)	www.ready.gov
U.S. Department of Health and Human Services	www.hhs.gov
U.S. Geological Survey (disasters/emergencies)	www.usgs.gov
WebMD	www.webmd.com
American Red Cross	www.redcross.org
Local Weather Web Site	_____

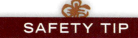

SAFETY TIP

Program the following numbers into your phone for quick and easy dialing of these important contacts.

Medical Emergencies

Call 911 for any medical emergency.

Poison Control Center	800-222-1222
National Suicide Prevention Lifeline	800-273-8255
Alcohol Drug Treatment Referrals (national)	800-996-3784
Centers for Disease Control (national)	800-232-4636
Nearest Hospital	Phone number: _____
Alternative Hospital	Phone number: _____
Detox Center	Phone number: _____
Drug Rehabilitation Clinic	Phone number: _____
Urgent Care Center	Phone number: _____
Medical Non-Emergencies	
Health Care Professionals and Consumers	800-358-9295
National AIDS Hotline	800-342-2437
County Health Offices	Phone number: _____
Cancer Care	800-813-4673
National Rosacea Society	888-NO-BLUSH or www.rosacea.org/index.php

American Acne & Rosacea Society   888-744-DERM or www.
                                         acnesociety.org

Physician   Phone number: _____
Physician (alternative)   Phone number: _____
Dermatologist (3 choices recommended)   Phone number: _____
Dermatologist 2   Phone number: _____
Dermatologist 3   Phone number: _____
Plastic Surgeon 1   Phone number: _____
Plastic Surgeon 2   Phone number: _____
Plastic Surgeon 3   Phone number: _____
Endocrinologist   Phone number: _____
Acupuncturist   Phone number: _____
Chiropractor   Phone number: _____
Pharmacist   Phone number: _____
Local CPR/First-Aid Training   Phone number: _____
Other Specialists   Phone number: _____
                                         Phone number: _____

Suppliers (support for problem resolution)
Name_____   Phone number: _____
Name_____   Phone number: _____
Name_____   Phone number: _____
Name_____   Phone number: _____
Name_____   Phone number: _____

Non-Medical Emergencies

Call 911 for any emergency where police are needed.
Emergency Broadcast System   800-237-3239
Local Radio Station (main)   Phone number: _____
Local Radio Station (alternative)   Phone number: _____
Local Television (main)   Phone number: _____
Local Television (alternative 1)   Phone number: _____
Local Television (alternative 2)   Phone number: _____
City Police (non-emergency)   Phone number: _____
County Police (non-emergency)   Phone number: _____
State Patrol (non-emergency)   Phone number: _____

Transportation

Evacuation Routes   _____
State Patrol   Phone number: _____
State Highway Weather Cams   http:// _____
State Road Conditions   Phone number: _____
Subway Service   Phone number: _____
Light Rail Service   Phone number: _____
Train Service   Phone number: _____
Bus Service   Phone number: _____
Taxi Service   Phone number: _____
Other   Phone number: _____

Abuse and Crime

Childhelp (national child abuse hotline)	800-422-4453
Police (nonemergency local number)	Phone number: _____
Child Protection Services	Phone number: _____
National Center for Victims of Crime	800-394-2255
National Domestic Violence Hotline	800-799-7233
Mental Health America	800-969-6642
Local Crisis Hotline	Phone number: _____
Mental Health Care Facility	Phone number: _____
Counselor(s)	Phone number: _____
	Phone number: _____

Accidents, Injuries, and Legal Action

OSHA:	800-321-OSHA (6742)
Incident Report Personnel:	Phone number: _____
Maintenance Personnel:	Phone number: _____
Landlord (for rental property)	Phone number: _____
Professional Insurance Firm:	Phone number: _____
Other Insurance:	Phone number: _____
Legal Representation:	Phone number: _____

ESTHETICS-RELATED CONTACTS

There are many contacts related to the esthetics profession. Provided for you is a listing of some of the more commonly used Web sites; you may list additional sites for your own locality or preferences.

Esthetics-Related Web Sites

Aesthetics International Association, www.aestheticsassociation.com

American Acne and Rosacea Society, www.acnesociety.org

American Academy of Micropigmentation, www.micropigmentation.org

Associated Bodywork and Massage Professionals, www.abmp.com/home/

Associated Skin Care Professionals, www.ascpskincare.com

Black Spa Professionals Association, www.orgsites.com/ca/b-spa/

California Spa Association, www.californiaspaassociation.com

CIDESCO International, www.cidesco.com

Day Spa Association, www.dayspaassociation.com

The Esthetician Channel, www.estheticianchannel.com

International Esthetician Association, www.aestheticsassociation.com

International Medical Spa Association (IMSA), www.dayspaassociation.com

International Spa Association, www.experienceispa.com

International Therapy Examination Council (ITEC), www.itec-usa.com or www.itecworld.co.uk

Las Vegas Spa Association, www.lvspas.com

National Aesthetic and Spa Network, www.nasnbiz.com

National Coalition of Estheticians, Manufacturers/Distributors and Associations, www.ncea.tv

National Institutes of Health, www.nih.gov

National Psoriasis Foundation, www.psoriasis.org

National Rosacea Society, www.rosacea.org

North Carolina Cosmetology Aesthetics Nails Association, www.nccan.org

Professional Beauty Association, www.probeauty.org

Salon and Spa Association, www.salonspaassociation.com

Society of Permanent Cosmetic Professionals, www.spcp.org

Society for Clinical and Medical Hair Removal, www.scmhr.org

Society of Dermatology SkinCare Specialists, www.sdss.tv

South Carolina Esthetics Association, www.scesthetics.org

Spa Industry Associations, www.spatrade.com

U.S. State Board of Cosmetology Listing, www.beautytech.com/st_boards.htm

Virginia State Association for Skin Care Professionals, www.vsascp.com

ESTHETICIAN'S GUIDE TO CLIENT SAFETY AND WELLNESS

Department of Health and Human Services, National Center for Immunization and Respiratory Diseases. (2011). ACIP recommendations. Atlanta, GA: Centers for Disease Control and Prevention. Retrieved from http://www.cdc.gov/vaccines/pubs/acip-list.htm

Hand Hygiene for Certified Lay Responders and the Lay Community Responder. (2006). ACFAS. Retrieved from http://www.instructorscorner.org/media/resources/SAC/Hand%20Hygiene%20for%20First%20Aid.pdf

Harrison, J. (2008). *Aromatherapy*. Clifton Park, NY: Delmar.

NCEA Code of Ethics. (n.d.). Retrieved from http://www.ncea.tv/positions/positions_code_ethics.html

Occupational Safety and Health Administration. (2001). Recording and reporting occupational injuries and illness (1904.39). Washington D.C.: U.S. Department of Labor. Retrieved from http://www.osha.gov/pls/oshaweb/owadisp.show_document?p_table=STANDARDS&p_id=12783

Schmaling, S. (2009). *A Comprehensive Guide to Equipment*. Clifton Park, NY: Delmar

Sudden Deaths from Cardiac Arrest—Statistics. (2004). Retrieved from http://www.americanheart.org/downloadable/heart/1103835297279FS27SDCA5.pdf

U.S. Department of Health and Human Services. (2003). Disclosures for public health activities (45 CFR 164.512(b)). Washington D.C.: Retrieved from http://www.hhs.gov/ocr/privacy/hipaa/understanding/special/publichealth/publichealth.pdf

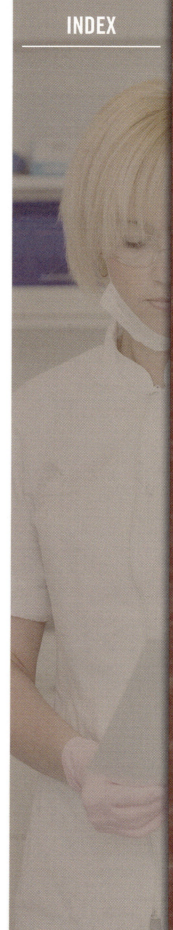